DR. DAVE HEPBURN

the DOCTOR IS IN(*sane*)

• • •

*Indispensable
Advice from Dr. Dave*

GREYSTONE BOOKS
D&M PUBLISHERS INC.
Vancouver/Toronto/Berkeley

.09 10 11 12 13   5 4 3 2 1

Greystone Books
A division of D&M Publishers Inc.
2323 Quebec Street, Suite 201
Vancouver BC Canada V5T 4S7
www.greystonebooks.com

Library and Archives Canada Cataloguing in Publication
Hepburn, David, 1958–
The doctor is in(sane) : indispensable advice from
Dr. Dave / David Hepburn.
Includes index.

ISBN 978-1-55365-408-7

1. Medicine—Humor. 2. Medicine, Popular. I. Title.
R705.H463 2009   610.2′07   C2008-906147-0

Editing by Kathy Sinclair
Cover photos by Tammy Doddis
Printed and bound in Canada by Friesens
Printed on acid-free paper that is forest friendly (100% post-consumer
recycled paper) and has been processed chlorine free
Distributed in the U.S. by Publishers Group West

The information contained in this book is not intended to serve as a replacement
for professional medical advice. Any use of the information in this book is at the reader's
discretion. The author and publisher specifically disclaim any and all liability from
the use or application of any information contained in this book. A health care
professional should be consulted regarding your specific condition.

The material in this book has been adapted from Dave Hepburn's
weekly column in the Unwind section of *The Province* (Vancouver).

We gratefully acknowledge the financial support of the Canada Council for the
Arts, the British Columbia Arts Council, the Province of British Columbia through
the Book Publishing Tax Credit, and the Government of Canada through the Book
Publishing Industry Development Program (BPIDP) for our publishing activities.

THE DOCTOR IS IN(SANE)

(*Contents*)

(*Introduction*)

THE CURE FOR WHAT AILS YOU

Being a doctor filled with wanderlust has taken me on some remarkable adventures and given me some splendid insights. I feel fortunate to have embraced a career that allows me to take drugs (so to speak), a stethoscope, and some barely used tongue depressors and go sweat like a sumo in the jungles of Vanuatu, cavort aboard a warship during the Persian Excursion, march into an Olympic stadium, and yes, even practice medicine in a more conventional role in hospitals and clinics.

But wherever I lay my size 7½ latex-free rubber gloves, I have practiced medicine with a touch of humor—perhaps, as has oft been suggested, because *I* am touched. As such, this book is a unique compilation of fascinating yet sound medical advice explained in a way that may well make you herniate something.

That being said, laughter is not the best medicine. Sorry, but no matter how hard I, as a physician, snicker and snort at a sagging sigmoid, hoot and holler at a hookworm, or chortle and chuckle at a charley horse, the problem gets no better. Healing requires hospitals in commotion and surgeons with notions, potions, more potions, and oceans of lotions, not a gaggle of gig-gling gigglers (eat your myocardium out, Seuss).

No, laughter is not the best medicine. *Medicine* is the best medicine. But that doesn't mean that doctors have to be dour, dreary, and mirthless. They can be like me: incompetent. I have discovered that a vast depth of incompetence can be covered up if a patient has a whopping good time. They lie there, thinking, "This guy with an arrow sticking out of his head is undoubtedly a buffoon, but I think I feel better." As one of my favorite philoso-pher fools, Willy Wonka, put it, "A little nonsense now and then is relished by the wisest men."

Famous clown-doctor Patch Adams, modeling a sartorial taste that resembled the result of a high-speed collision between Krusty the Clown and Elton John, once looked me in the eye and said, "Dave, you're standing on my freakin' foot," followed by a kinder, gentler, "You need to realize that humor and fun are two of the greatest antidotes to human pain and suffering. Now please get off my foot." His size 28 clown shoes were hard not to stand on, but they remain very hard to fill. Before long he even had me smelling the water lily in his lapel. Now I wear one.

I have realized that Patch Adams is right. Learning is better when you're having fun. Teaching is better when you're having fun. And yes, even being ill is better when you're inclined to see the funnier side of life. Laughter, it turns out, is hazardous to your illness.

When I graduated medical school, the dean took me aside and said, "Son, first of all, don't ever let me catch you practicing on my family. Second, remember that 50 per cent of what you have learned is right and 50 per cent is wrong. Problem is, we don't know which 50 is which. Now go out and practice." And I have come to find out he was right. Medicine is such a dynamic field that it changes seemingly by the nanosecond.

By the time your retinas hungrily scan the words on these pages, the treatment for head lice may be a single pill from moss grown only on the sunny side of the Tasmanian tea tree during kookaburra mating season—or perhaps it will simply remain a blowtorch. Heart attacks might be cured by an antibiotic that Fleming forgot was brewing in the lint of his pants pocket.

By taking a drop of blood and running it through a biochip we might soon be able to predict illnesses that rest in your genes. Then, hopefully we can prevent you from ever getting these diseases by putting you in quarantine until, say, George Clooney and Hugh Laurie come up with a cure. But in the meantime, this is as good as it gets.

As I travel the world learning, teaching, and speaking, I am always thrilled to discover that the cure for what ails you (or what will soon ail you) may include the new, exciting, highly advanced technological diagnostics and treatments evolving in research centers and tertiary care hospitals.

Then again, it may simply involve . . . a good hoot.

KICKING

(DEATH *in the*)

HEAD

DUMBBELLS
Meet my eldest son.
Age: 18
Height: 6'1"
Weight: 190 lbs.
Occupation: Hockey player
IQ: Hockey player
Physique: Muscular, as in tossing opposing players through boards.
Favorite novel: *Horton Hears a Who*
Favorite cuisine: "Quizzing??? I don't like quizzes."

"DAD, THE BOYS and I were talking on the bus on the way to the game. Somebody asked if anyone thought they could take out their dads." (Please note: "take out" in this instance doesn't mean taking Dad out to the Chinese takeout, but rather is hockey-ese for "flatten.") "Not one guy on the team thinks he could take his dad. But if I could, I would do it LIKE THIS!"

As he lunges to grab my knees, I deflect him with my love handles. But he grabs one of my chins and flings me toward the couch.

"Easy, boy, I'd hate to break your... oh look, your uvula is showing!" As he checks his body for a part of his anatomy that might be embarrassingly exposed, I sneak off to the phone.

"Hello, personal trainer, I need to get stronger. I've noticed that my son bench presses 230 pounds in our garage gym. I attempted the same, only to require an emergency barbellectomy from my nipples. Obviously, when it comes to dumbbells, I'm a big one. Should I really be weight training at my age?"

"Without a doubt," the trainer replied. "Don't wait to do weights. Strength training is an important part of establishing great health. A well-looked-after set of muscles not only makes the body stronger and more physically capable but can also prevent several illnesses, at any age."

"Such as?"

"Well, if you allow your muscles to deteriorate, your joints begin to rot, a condition known as osteoarthritis, which plagues about 30 million North Americans. By toning muscle, you decrease the wear and tear on your knees, hips, and back. For example, a simple 20 per cent increase in strength in your thigh muscles can decrease knee problems by half."

"Speaking of 'osteo,' what about..."

"Osteoporosis? Absolutely. Osteoporosis victims fill orthopedic wards across the country. Their hips and backs turn to chalk and crumble. Weight training, also known as resistance training, can increase bone density, particularly in the hips. Those who begin muscle strengthening early in life can thwart degenerating bone diseases later on. In fact, many infirmities associated with old age are simply a result of muscle wasting and imbalance. So hurry up and weight."

The trainer cleared his uvula and continued. "Strong muscles will also decrease body fat, lower fats swilling about the bloodstream, increase basal metabolic rate, and can actually strengthen another rather important muscle—heart muscle. Another by-product of a good strengthening program is being physically better able to go out and tackle any sport, from mud wrestling to ballroom dancing."

"I'm not sure I want to dance with some girl with biceps bigger than mine."

"Knowing you, that would limit your opportunities. But in fact, women do not bulk up with resistance training. Instead, they lose fat and gain lean body mass. They tone their muscles, subsequently developing better coordination and agility."

"Well, I prefer dancing with girls with two left feet anyway. That way, we move in unison."

"My advice, if you want to grow muscle sprouts, is to start low and go slow," warned the trainer. "But it is best to first consult an expert in order to avoid wrecking yourself. Resistance training must be individualized. In your case, for example, you'll need to figure out which chin to chin up."

WALK A DOG, SAVE A LIFE

Every morning I am forced to walk my border collie/lab/ADHD cross, who wakes me up at the crack of dawn by placing a wet nose or raspy tongue on any part of my crack-of-dawn anatomy that happens to be extending over the edge of the bed. Should, at the time, I happen to be in dreamland, protecting my rhinoceros farm against a flock of savage Beanie Babies while wearing only golf cleats, her well-placed snout will cause me to bolt straight up in bed, frightening off all Beanies and rhinos. This seems to please her immensely, judging by the dance of joy she performs, beating to shreds everything in reach of her tail and dragging me out for her walkies.

While I stumble outside, barely able to open my eyes, she zips and spins about as if she's spent the night lapping Red Bull from the toilet. We plod up the road to the park, where we greet other drowsy dog owners with a groggy hello and a quick sniff. The dogs greet each other as well. But as I reach my house again

I, at least, appreciate that I have already undertaken a third of the ten thousand steps that I, and every one of you, need to take every day.

I have a friend who has been a letter carrier forever and has been trim and slim as a result of his active job of losing mail and pepper-spraying rottweilers.

But he retired last year and, lo and behold, much to my sedentary pleasure, a wee pot has formed just above his belt line. I am overjoyed.

As a result of the car, computer, and cable, we have become a supersized sedentary society. I asked several patients to guesstimate the number of steps they took in a day based on standards I gave them. Then they used a pedometer and were shocked to know how sedentary their lives really were. Ten thousand steps (roughly five miles) is the equivalent of fifty pounds a year of calorie burn. Search "10,000 steps" to find many websites that will show you how to take these steps. Of course, if you need a website to learn how to walk, then apparently you might need the Twelve-Step site first.

A recent study from the hold-the-Mayo Clinic found that obese folks (those with a BMI greater than 33) spent an average of 2 hours a day longer sitting than their leaner counterparts. Though both groups were found to lie down for the same amount of time, obese people sat for an average of 9.5 hours a day, expending 350 fewer calories! That adds up to 36 pounds a year for plunking your Kentucky-Fried Krispy-Kremed keyster at a keyboard or a Kia for an extra 2 hours a day.

Our routine energy expenditure is known as Non Exercise Activity Thermogenesis, or NEAT. This term describes how active we are when we're not exercising. Those with low NEAT often complain of having "low metabolism," when in fact they just feel a need to spend more time sitting. Those with higher NEAT may actually have a difference in their brain chemicals that requires them to sit less. If they also happen to have three nostrils and a tail, they would be classified NEAT freaks.

So, to avoid being labeled sedentary, take ten thousand steps every day in *addition* to your exercise program, and sit less than 7.5 hours. Add up the difference and you will lose eighty-six pounds per year, and therefore disappear altogether in three years. If you need help getting started, you can borrow my rhino disturber.

GET WAISTED

"Good to see you too, doctor, but, umm, why are you wrapping your arms around my waist?"

"Actually I can't quite, so I'm going to attach this measuring tape to the post and have you spin around."

"What does it read?"

"Forty-six."

"Which is what, in inches?"

"Okay. Now I have to measure your hip-to-waist ratio. That would be both hips, Bloggins."

"Whoa! I'll bring flowers next time, doc."

FORGET THOSE PASSÉ BMI numbers. It turns out that those calculations were useless, corrupt, and irrelevant, the Chicago Cubs of measurements. Yesterday's mistake. By taking the square root of your height minus your weight on Thursday and multiplying it by the third power of the log of your dandruff count, you could determine your BMI (Body Mass Ice cream). This was apparently a predictor of your cardiac risk.

One of my small Asian buddies, Vietnamese by ethnicity, would taunt me by sneaking up behind me as though I were Peter Sellers, and reach around me to start chest compressions. Even though he had a bit of a sake gut himself, his BMI was considered low, and he would tend to laud it over us Caucasian behemoths. If I were bigger and had a meaner streak I would've sat on the little pest. Meanwhile, my rugby player patients had BMIs that, according to the charts, meant that they should have had seventeen heart attacks, thirty-four strokes, and sung the lead for

Aida. Fact is, they didn't have an ounce of fat on them outside of their skulls. A BMI does not differentiate muscle from fat from bone from Cheeze Doodles.

The waist-hip ratio has now been determined to be the most accurate predictor of our risk of having the Big Mac Attack, and now for scientific reasons.

Big, bulging bellies store a nasty fat that produces nasty hormones that do nasty things to the heart. Belly fat clogs up the liver, messes up insulin regulation, and changes cholesterol levels for the worse.

1. Put down this book and go and find a measuring tape.
2. Pick up this book to read the next instruction.
3. Take your belly girth. Quit sucking in! Take it just above your navel (after removing all lint).
4. Hmmm. Put down the book and go and find a longer tape.
5. Okay, now try the hips. Measure about the widest part of your caboose, the part that picks up the chair when you stand up.
6. Get son's calculator. Divide the waist by the hip.

Should you have a ratio over 0.90 for men or 0.85 for women, then you are apple-shaped. You apples get primarily waisted with your fat storage and are in some metabolic trouble. You are predisposed to diabetes, heart attack, cancer, and hypertension, and may end up an apple crumble. Fat around your belly means you have fat around your vital organs.

But if your ratio is less than 0.72, i.e., fat predominantly in your hips, then you are pear-shaped. Those who are tragically hip with their fat storage have a difficult time shedding this type of fat, even though it is safer to have fat on your hips than on your belly.

"But doc, I think I'm a watermelon."

"You know, I think you're right, Bloggins. Here, meet my little buddy from Hanoi."

RESISTING RESISTANCE

Every year, the church I attend holds a "friendly" Strong Man competition. This social spectacle held in the church parking lot draws a huge crowd and several ambulances. Now behold, last year I was verily humiliated at the event; yea, I was brought down to the depths of testosterone hell with a less-than-saintly effort. But this year I repented of my sedentary ways by weight training, and so was hoping for more celestial results. The ten competitors were a pious bunch, including the likes of defending champion Dirty Dave Watters, Sister Robbie Cossette, and Marty (Samson) Kinnear.

The first event was the truck pull. A rope was attached to the truck and a harness to my chest. The whistle blew and I strained at the harness, which only served to make my belly jut out like that of a woman about to give birth to a flock of sumo wrestlers. Despite the brake being left on (according to my lawyer), I came in eighth.

The next event, the drum lift, required the lifting of truck drums weighing, I believe, just under 47,000 tons each. I won this event by tossing the drums up on a platform after warning other competitors of the excruciating pain involved in hernia operations.

The pew toss was almost canceled due to excessive gum. Third place, but sore.

The anvil lift involved repetitive power squatting and lifting of the world's heaviest anvil. The number to beat was now eleven, set by Nasty Neil Watters, brother to the defending champion, DNA results pending. I grunted out twelve reps and most of my pelvic floor.

I hobbled into the final event, a brutal obstacle course of chains and rocks, tied for the lead with the defending champ.

Many theories exist on resistance training, including the theory of many of my patients that it is best to resist training altogether. But weight training is so vitally important to overall health that, well, I'm writing about it.

Who should weight train?
- youth
- elderly
- everyone in between

Benefits of lifting weights range from the obvious to the startling. Recently it has been shown that, by increasing muscle density through weight training, insulin acts much more effectively. In other words, lifting a few weights every week might prevent prediabetics (which in North America is apparently most of us) from going completely sugary. It could also replace or reduce the need for some medications in diabetics.

Weight training also helps:
- lower blood lipids.
- decrease the risk of falls, so dangerous in the elderly.
- reduce the risk of developing osteoporosis. Weight training is a major part of any osteoporosis prevention program.
- fight osteoarthritis. Toned muscles means less strain on the joints.
- turn that flabdomen into a washboard. By increasing muscle density, the basal metabolic rate rises, more calories are burned every day, and abdominal fat is shed. Comparable to turning your locomotor system from a weak four-cylinder to a fuel burning v-8 engine. They don't call them muscle cars for nothing.
- strengthen the heart and lower resting blood pressure. While resistance training strengthens skeletal muscle and aerobic exercise strengthens the heart, weight training indirectly improves the entire cardiovascular system.
- foster a sense of well-being. I personally find that being ripped is infinitely more fun as I now strut the beach kicking sand with abandon rather than with an abdomen.
- win strong-man competitions at church, daycare, or quilting bees.

Sedentary people lose 10 per cent of their muscle mass per decade after age thirty. Thus, regardless of your age, I strongly suggest you hurry up and weight. It is absolutely essential for great health. Start low and go slow, but get started and lift weights twice a week.

By the way, pending urine test results, I am now the church champ. In thy face, brethren!

KICKING DEATH IN THE HEAD

A Montreal woman recently developed a somewhat rare and fascinating condition. She has been practicing yoga for years and can now contort and fold her body into positions that would give my hernias hernias. She can bend over and slap her palms on the floor while touching her forehead to her knees. She also walks quicker than the average man and talks faster than the average woman. She flits about as though she exists on a diet of lemon rinds and Red Bull. Do not enter into a battle of wits with this woman—you will lose. If repartee was a sword fight, you would be sliced, diced, and iced, and then the pieces would be tossed with relish upon the scrap heap of past victims. When her phone rings she traverses the room in an instant and answers it before the first ring has ended. She can recite baseball stats with such detail and accuracy that she can tell you how many hits, runs, scratches, and spits each ballplayer has. Recently, a police cruiser went to her home and carted her off to help her deal with this unusual condition. They were taking her to a celebration of her one hundredth birthday.

She is my great aunt Gertie, she is my GREAT aunt Gertie. She has not just survived or crept up to the century mark; this feisty, pint-sized bull terrier has crashed through that barrier like my stocks crash through record lows. She is brighter now than I will ever be, sprier than spring, and she is laughing and chuckling her way past one hundred as though it were twenty. When she takes me for a hike up the boulevard, she leaves me behind, choking in the clouds of smoke that stream off her Air Jordans.

Her brother lived to ninety-nine, her sisters (who included the most wonderful woman to ever set foot on this planet, my grandmother) lived into their late nineties. Genes being what they are, I may yet get to see President George Z. Bush.

How rare is this condition? Of every 5,129 people born in North America, only one will reach age one hundred. Few will blow by it the way Gertie has.

Some families possess the longevity gene, located somewhere on chromosome 4, that offers prolonged protection from age-related diseases. One American family had five of seven children live to be centenarians. One brother blew out his 108th birthday candles in the presence of his 102- and 101-year-old younger sisters. Remarkably, many of these centenarians don't simply survive to 100; they are in strikingly good shape, mentally and physically robust, particularly those from families in which living long is the norm. Oddly enough, most seem to share a sense of fun and a sense of curiosity—perhaps a trait of this Ponce de León gene, or perhaps just a trait that makes longevity enjoyable. They look and act much younger than the average person of similar age. I, for example, have been told I act quite a bit a younger than I actually am. Apparently my mature years are still a long way in front of in of me yet.

North America currently is home to about 75,000 centenarians, 30 per cent of whom live independently and claim to be in excellent health. Another 40 per cent claim to be in good health. They have escaped the big three: stroke, cancer, and heart attacks, which normally ravage those in their forties to seventies. Chances are that if you have avoided these crippling killers by age ninety, then you have avoided them altogether. You get to die of some other cause like pneumonia or a bungee-jumping accident. Assuming you don't sabotage your genetic predisposition by smoking, drinking, or driving behind Gertie in downtown Montreal, then expect to live to your family's age (do your genealogy and you'll know exactly what your life expectancy is).

Seventy-five per cent of today's centenarians are women, likely due to the stress-free life that we men allow them to enjoy.

As I left this Montreal party, my great-aunt, who stood part-way down a staircase, stretched out her leg at an impossible angle and rested it on my shoulder,

"I hope to see you next year for your 101st party," I placated.

She snapped back, "Why? Are you sick?"

Gertie—she's a beaut.

THE SKINNY ON LAWN BOWLERS

"Rumors of rampant use of steroids among the lawn bowlers has me concerned. Apparently steroids and soup causes Polident to lose its grip.

"So to the rowers I say, keep on stroking,

To the hockey players, keep on scoring top shelf,

To the cyclists, keep on pedaling,

To the lawn bowlers. . . keep on breathing."

—excerpts from a speech given by Dr. Hepburn at a major sports awards banquet

THESE COMMENTS brought upon me the collective wrath of the lawn bowling grandternity. Walkers shook violently, pacemakers seized up, and hearing aids began shrieking all over the room. Letters of complaint began to pile up in my rather expansive "hate-mail in-box," accompanied by ticking cupcakes and cyanide-laced brownies.

"How could you, as a hockey player, the intellectual giants of sport, take potshots at the lawn bowlers."

"You have sent the lawn bowling movement back centuries." (No doubt verified by several of the charter members.)

"Your mother. . ."

I had been well and truly chastised, and as it turns out, deservedly so.

"I challenge you to try to lawn bowl," came a final admonition. *"You'd be amazed at the skill it takes."*

And I was! While out cycling one day, I happened upon a lawn bowling yard or pit or quilting bee or whatever it is and paused to watch. Fearing I'd be recognized and beaten with canes, I went home, put on my, er. . . a skirt and some lipstick, and returned in disguise. I was amazed at the accuracy with which these players could bowl a heavy ball across a lawn and have it curve, spin, and stop on a dime (or possibly it was a tooth). While more and more young people are discovering the fun of lawn bowling, it does remain a sport dominated by older players. That said, doctors have all seen eighty-five-year-old patients who are significantly younger than some sixty-five-year-olds. These lawn bowlers certainly fit that category. They are an active, bustling, happy, and evidently healthy bunch. The camaraderie and laughter was a genuine pleasure to observe as I wiped the mascara from my face. Seldom did I hear anything like "Mildred, in your dentures, baby!" I was also impressed that among the men who were lawn bowling, there were no fat guys. Though the women outnumbered the men five to one, the men were all slim, trim, and fit. It struck me that not only do obese men not play sports, they don't live long enough to be able to.

A wealth of data now exists that proves that exercising leads to significantly improved quality and quantity of life for the elderly. Group exercising, much more successful than solo home exercising, reduces depression and joint pain, and the risk of diabetes, heart disease, and those dreaded falls. Exercise increases strength and improves body composition by decreasing fat while increasing lean body mass. Astonishingly, 42 per cent of those aged sixty to sixty-nine are obese, as are 35 per cent of those between seventy and seventy-nine and 19 per cent over eighty. The obese generally don't make it into their eighties. Frailty is the natural result of deconditioning, the disuse of muscles and metabolism. Exercise can often prevent the vicious circle of frailty → disuse → illness → frailty.

Three different types of exercises should be incorporated into the lives of seniors: strength training, aerobic activity, and balance training such as tai chi. Before starting a program, see a doctor who knows how to write exercise prescriptions (not all do), and then start low and go slow.

On behalf of my granny, who accidentally forgot to send me a Christmas present after my speech, I suggest that when you really get fit, agile, forgiving, athletic, strong, forgiving, intelligent, forgiving, and beautiful, you might be ready to start... lawn bowling.

DIE YOUNG . . . AT AN OLD AGE

BLOGGINS, Cecil—passed away suddenly at the age of 173 in a bungee-jumping accident. Predeceased by Cheryl (née Neigh), his wife of 138 years. Survived by 4 children, 14 grandchildren, 54 great grandchildren, 287 great-great grandchildren, 792 great-great-great grandchildren, 2175 great-great-great-great grandchildren, and a small town of great-great-great-great-great grandchildren. Cecil was born naturally in 2003 in East San Diego (formerly called Phoenix). He is a survivor of the Bush dynasty and the earthquake of '09. Cecil's mammoth home runs will be missed by the boys of the Overtimers Ball Team. In lieu of flowers, please send donations to Chicago Cubs Pennant Assistance program. Cecil's one regret was that he didn't live long enough to see the Cubs win it all. In fact, Cecil's dying words were, "I still don't understand why they traded four first-round picks for that eighty-seven-year-old catcher. Sure, he had a lot of years left, but..." Cecil was a successful artificial intelligence mechanic as a youth but after a midlife crisis at the age of ninety-one, he returned to college. He graduated with a degree in azimuthal biomolecular tectonics and began his own discount organ-cloning company. Funeral will be held on Saturday at Lincoln Stadium, right after the game.

IS AGING A DISEASE? Hmmm. Consider some of the physical "symptoms" of aging: heart failure, kidney failure, hair loss, skin thinning, brain atrophy, osteoporosis, prostatic hypertrophy, sweater vests, cataracts, hearing loss, and immune deficiency. Sound like a disease? If so, can it be beaten?

According to the AAAAM (American Association of Anti-Aging Medicine), not only is aging a disease, but it is often a fatal one. They feel that medicine spends excessive energy, talent, and money in treating the outcomes of aging rather than preventing many of the problems that manifest later in life. A4M searches not only for ways to prolong life span, but for ways to increase *health* span. In 1900 the average life expectancy was 48 years. A century later it has risen to 76 in America, 80 in Japan, and close to 106 in the population of Ford Escort car drivers who precede me at each stoplight when I'm in a hurry. The lifespan for following generations is projected by some to be 125!

We die of aging because various cells of various important organs die. Can pre-programmed cell death (called apoptosis) be delayed or even halted? Already, researchers have been able to extend the life span of fruit flies and lab rats by four times! (Thanks for nothing.)

Dr. Ronald Klatz, president of A4M, speculates, "Medical knowledge is doubling every three years. With advances in genetic engineering, organ transplantation, and molecular machines, we will see life expectancy jump from seventy-seven to eighty-five in the next ten years and then steadily increasing from there." Further commenting on conquering cell death and disease, he makes this astonishing prediction: "Soon we'll be running out of reasons to die. Heart disease and diabetes will be eliminated in ten years, Alzheimer's in fifteen, and cancer will be cured in twenty years. By the year 2047 the leading causes of death will be accidents, homicide, and suicide, particularly among Cubs fans." Okay, I added the last phrase, but I assume that if we are all living that long, that robustly, that disease-free, then the term "die-hard fan" will take on a whole new meaning. "Pro" wrestling's *Smack Down* will be a family affair.

So what are we supposed to do now, as we wade through the cusp of this biomolecular revolution? Are you preparing, physically and mentally, to live a longer life than your grandparents did? As the science of youthful aging is further advanced, we are admonished to adhere to the principles of healthy living that we know all too well. Maximize your exercise; smoke and you croak; fill up with fruits, veggies, and grains to preserve your heart, liver, and brains; don't make alcohol your last call; reduce the weight or you reduce the wait (for angioplasty).

As Mickey Mantle stated, "If I'd known I was going to live this long, I would have taken better care of myself." As Mickey Mouse stated, "Wow, I'm immortal!" And as anti-aging researcher Dr. Ivan Popov stated, "Wouldn't it be great if we all died young. . . late in life."

GOOD GUANO

"Doctor, I'd like to know if any of these supplements are interfering with the prescription you gave me for my foot fungus."

"What's the problem, Bloggins?"

"Well, I've noticed my left pancreas is itchy and my hair is sluggish."

"Exactly what supplements are you taking?"

"Not sure, so I brought them with me." At this time I often hear a loud beeping sound, as if a large delivery truck were backing up, whereupon I glance outside to observe a large delivery truck backing up. Out tumbles the prize products of infomercials, *National Enquirer* ads, and so-called "health shows" (the ones that exhibit every health expert with the exception of actual health experts).

"Here they are. Let's see." As Bloggins begins stacking bottles upon plastic bottles of virgin beaver tooth extract and beta609 isoelbowanoids, I note a preponderance of items beginning with G, such as ginseng, ginkgo, grapeseed, assorted green thingama-jigs, and giblets of Gary Gilmore. As Bloggins proudly looks over his small pharmacy of assorted supplements, I soon learn that he has no idea what they are actually for.

"By the way, do you take any supplements, doctor?"

"I do."

"What?" he asks, eager to add whatever I might suggest to his little armada of bottles.

"Well, on a daily basis I take a Snickers pill, but when the moon is exactly one-third full, I take a couple of Skittles, particularly if I feel my serum trans fats are getting a little low."

But I actually *do* take supplements. My constant perusal of *The Lancet, New England Journal of Medicine,* and *Vogue* has convinced me to take curcumin and salmon oil. I need supplements to make up for the paucity of these essential nutrients at the grocery store I usually shop at, the HersheySnickers Market.

As I enjoy expanding voluminously on the benefits of salmon (for previous references please contact the Pulitzer archives and mention my name repeatedly), I turn my attention now to curcumin, as many of you do if someone has just ingested a bowl of curry before invading your private space. Curcumin is the component of the turmeric spice that gives curry its brilliant color and pungency. My mother once made hot curried chicken when I was six, and I'm convinced that the part I didn't toss to the regretful dog is still eating away at my olfactory glands.

Curcumin has previously been touted to increase our brainpower, improve our vision, and give us happier prostates, apparently for good reasons. It has excellent antioxidant, anti-inflammatory, and antiamyloid properties. (Nasty amyloids are constantly being implicated in Alzheimer's disease.) India has significantly less Alzheimer's than North America, to say nothing of a cancer rate ten times lower and a statistically significant lower number of Alanis Morissette fans. Could curcumin be the reason Indians are so much healthier? It is currently being tested in multiple studies as a chemotherapeutic or chemopreventative agent because of its positive effects against cancer growth and spread. It is being studied in large, prestigious cancer centers for its antioxidant properties and is now being looked at for specific cancer prevention and even treatment, including the dangerous melanomas (moles gone wild). In one study, it caused melanoma cells to actually self-destruct.

Curcumin is very safe and tolerable in that ingesting bushels of this stuff appears to cause no toxicity whatsoever, unless the consumer is out on a first date. As more and more disease processes appear to depend on inflammation to wreak their havoc on our brains, arteries, and joints, curcumin offers us a safe and effective anti-inflammatory agent.

"Thanks, doc. You've convinced me. I'll go pick up some Skittles right away."

ONE HUNDRED WAYS TO
ENJOY LIVING TO ONE HUNDRED

To help patient patients remain patient while waiting to be a patient, I use a few distraction techniques out in the wailing room. I scatter about several *War and Peace* novels, scratch-and-sniff Rubik's dodecahedrons, and my son's *Where's Waldo* picture books (he still thinks his college roommate stole them).

I also hang a poster that generates no small amount of discussion, often spawning debates and even pitched battles involving syringes, rubber gloves, and the occasional broadsword. My patients used to say that if I ever wrote a book, this poster should be in it. So to all of you who waited seventeen hours to be seen for that saber slash, I dedicate this. Hope you make it to one hundred.

1. Don't worry about the future
2. Or fret about the past
3. Wear your seat belt

4. Walk a dog in the morning
5. Take the stairs
6. Be curious
7. Avoid smokers
8. Watch what you eat
9. Watch what you say
10. Don't talk with your mouth full
11. Get a massage
12. Ski
13. Make time
14. Make children
15. Make time for children
16. Do crosswords
17. Avoid cross words
18. Forgive
19. Be an optimist
20. Discover romance
21. Exercise every single day
22. Do tai chi
23. Plant a garden
24. Eat it
25. Cook with turmeric
26. Marry your sweetheart
27. Enjoy being single
28. Relax
29. Laugh easily
30. Lawn bowl
31. Do nothing in excess
32. Do everything in excess
33. Do chicken noodle soup on cold days
34. Make time for friends
35. Make new friends
36. Write an old friend
37. Get a flu shot

38. Reduce the carbs
39. Know your cholesterol levels
40. Do two outrageous things every year
41. Reduce calories
42. Learn to love what you see in the mirror
43. Sing in a choir
44. Sing in a car
45. Pamper yourself once a day
46. Carpe diem
47. Take setbacks with a smile, then forget them
48. Cuddle
49. Use olive oil
50. Be part of your community
51. Buy lemonade from kids
52. Eat broccoli
53. Take care of your bones
54. Be awestruck by lightning
55. Avoid being struck by lightning
56. Vacation vacation vacation
57. Take a long soak in a wide tub
58. Go to the country fair
59. Meditate
60. Eat fish often
61. Go fishing often
62. Spoil your grandchildren
63. Avoid supermodels
64. Build super models
65. Play an instrument
66. Power walk to the mall
67. Wrestle with kids
68. Grow flowers
69. Smell flowers
70. Socialize on weekends
71. Take long weekends
72. Write a poem

73. Walk in the woods
74. Check your blood pressure
75. Floss
76. Get rid of cable TV, except when it's time to. . .
77. Watch the play-offs
78. Contribute to charity
79. Play board games
80. Avoid mind games
81. Volunteer
82. Go to the movies
83. Don't rest on your laurels
84. Rest on a soft couch
85. Read in bed
86. Lift weights
87. Stretch your joints
88. Visit the elderly
89. Kiss a dog
90. Get up early, retire early
91. Read the classics
92. Read the comics
93. Debate stuff
94. Feed birds
95. Mess about in boats
96. Worship
97. Have your prostate and/or breasts checked
98. Learn to love your job, even your boss
99. Practice exactly what you preach
100. Listen to your doctor

GET

$$(\quad a \quad)$$

GRIPPE

WAX IN, WAX OUT

"*Whaaaad* he say, Mildred?"

"HE SAID YOU'RE DEAF, YOU OLD FOOL."

"I'm dead?"

"NO, BERT... NOT YET."

I finally interrupt this romantic interlude: "Mrs. Bloggins, your husband's ears are jammed with wax."

"I got jam on my slacks?" yells Bert.

Warning: If reading about bodily fluids makes you at all queasy, or if the phrase "bodily fluids" itself induces violent waves of nausea, perhaps you'd best not read this at the dinner table. In fact, it is foolish to ever read medical advice in the vicinity of tomato soup, cauliflower, refried beans, or sushi.

Today, EARWAX (retch).

Earwax, medically referred to as cerumen, has been tenderly cultured in your ear canal by Mother Nature for a reason... so leave it alone! (For those of you hard of hearing... SO LEAVE IT ALONE!) It is not bad stuff. It is good stuff. Cerumen is made by special glands called "plugger-uppers" that live on the outer third of your ear canal. Its sluggish existence has three purposes.

First, it protects the very sensitive skin of your ear canal from water and infections. Second, it protects your eardrum from dirt and grit by trapping it before it gets to the drum. Third, cerumen finds great glee in driving usually intelligent people to distraction as they attempt to roto-root it out with everything ranging from Q-tips to cue sticks.

If wax is so good for us, why do we try so hard to get it out? Perhaps it is a teleological obsession that began when mother Eve wet the corner of her fig leaf with saliva and ramrodded it down Cain's canal to get out the wax put there, no doubt, by the serpent. Or perhaps we have an innate desire to scrape off anything that isn't nailed to our carcass. Unfortunately, the practice of ramming bobby pins, fingernails, or darning needles into our ears is highly detrimental. Not only does it denude the ear of the protective cerumen and introduce microcracks into the skin of the canal itself (which, in turn, gets infected), but it also jams the wax up against a very flimsy eardrum. What follows: deafness, infection, swelling, itchiness, and pain in the canal that makes you rush down to the doctor with what is actually called "Q-tip ear." NEVER STICK ANYTHING SMALLER THAN YOUR ELBOW IN YOUR EAR!!

Warning: It seems that for every orifice in the human body, there is a "practitioner" willing to cleanse or irrigate it. The ear canal, unfortunately, is not immune. Ear candling is one of those ancient Druid practices invented by Charla Tan whereby the victim actually has hollow wax candles stuck in each ear, and then lit. The practitioner then dashes out of the room collapsing in spasms of laughter, sobered only by the fact that he or she has just made another fifty dollars. The candling creates a vacuum, wherein some earwax, along with significant amounts of cerebral gray matter, are sucked into the hollow tube.

While some folks generate a meager amount of wax, others make enough to plug up the entire canal . . . in Panama. In some cases, the natural process of wax removal does not work well, and the ear jams up. Avoid Q-tips at all costs. But before going to the doctor, please apply a few drops of olive or mineral oil or WD40 to the ear canal for three days, or mix baking soda with a couple of ounces of water and dump that in there three times a day for a couple of days. Then see the doctor, who will (retch... gag) gently flush your ear using a 300,000 psi power washer. The water is fired into your ear, where it strikes your drum and returns with the hated wax, unless, of course, you happen to watch a lot of Jerry Springer, in which case it comes flying out the other ear.

And then there's ol' Bert, who winks at me as he glances at Mildred and whispers, "Doc, just leave it in there."

GET A GRIPPE

Q. How can I differentiate a cold from the flu?

A. A cold is not as dramatic as the flu. The flu hits hard and fast. One moment you're dancing the tango with George Hamilton and the next, like many men forced to view *Dancing with the Stars*, you're begging for a quick death. Your fever is more intense than with a cold, your muscles and joints ache, and you become light-headed. Along with this you may get all the usual cold symptoms that everyone nose so well. With the flu, you don't want to get out of bed. With a cold, you want to get out of bed and strangle the person who came to your office with a cold looking for a miraculous cure that apparently nobody but your doctor has discovered.

Q. Can we catch a cold from spending too long in the cold?

A. We can't catch a cold from the cold any more than we can catch the flu from having flown.

Q. How can I avoid the flu?

A. The best way to avoid getting sick is to not breathe. Specifically, do not breathe the respiratory droplets of others around you who are teeming in viruses. Do not touch stuff that sick people touch, like pharmacy doorknobs, toilet levers, Jimmy Swaggart, aisle six at Costco, or grade 3 schoolteachers. WASH YOUR HANDS as though you suffer from obsessive-compulsive disorder. Wash for twenty seconds at a time. And, of course, get a flu shot.

Q. But the flu shot could possibly make me sick.

A. The only way you can catch the flu from the flu shot is if the flu shotter has a case of the flu and then coughs and sneezes all over the flu shotee while giving the shot.

Q. What about supplements to prevent cold and flu?

A. You should buy all the cold supplements advertised to the easily swayed. You will be left with no disposable income and, hence, won't be able to go shopping at Costco or touch Jimmy Swaggart.

Q. What's the best way to treat the flu/cold?

A. Chicken soup is as good as it gets, unless, of course, you're the chicken. The best you can do is treat the symptoms. For aches in your muscles and joints, use ibuprofen. For a stuffy nose, take a decongestant. Antibiotics are useless for either cold or flu and end up doing nothing but giving you a yeast infection some-where in a crevice or crease in your body that you wish yeast wouldn't find. If you catch the flu early, there are a couple of antiviral agents that might lessen the duration and the severity of the flu in some people. So it may be worthwhile to see a doc-tor in the very first hours after you have been belted by the flu. But if you have a cold, stay away from my freakin' office. Get a grippe. . . Okay, so you have a grippe, but I do not wish to catch your cold, no, I do not, Sam I am. Go see a reflexologist or Rich-ard Simmons. I'm sure they have a cure. I have no cure. Hey, if you've got a thirty-pound hernia dragging off the floor or a Doberman attached to your adrenals or an aorta about to bust, then great, I'd love to see you. But if you come with a cold, then all you will do is give me the cold and I will be forced to leave the office to go and see my doctor.

NO SNIVELING

"Son," I announced, turning to my twelve-year-old slumped in his seat in a when-will-we-get-there pose, "I want to stop in this next town and show you the greatest sign ever posted in sports arenas anywhere." He probably thought I was losing my few remaining marbles when we pulled into the tiny dry gulch town of Ashcroft, about two hundred miles from Vancouver, Canada. Having been impressed by this sign while playing in a hockey tournament many years earlier, I was eager to teach him a cardinal rule of life (hockey, of course, is life). We pulled up to the Drylands Arena only to find the rink locked up tighter than a jar of pickles. But on our tiptoes, as we peered through the glass of the door, we glimpsed the sign stretching in all its glory across the width of the rink. "NO SNIVELING."

"See that, boy? That is a great motto to live by when playing sports and when playing life." I glanced sideways at him, noting a concerned, quizzical look on his wee mug. Finally, looking up at me as though I'd taken one too many pucks to the noodle, he asked, "But Dad, what if they have a cold and just can't help it?"

After explaining the difference between sniffling and sniveling (though one often leads to the other), I realized that I could treat you, discerning and intelligent reader, to a complete synopsis of the causes, concerns, and treatment of a drippy snout.

Besides the usual colds, grippes, and tax seasons, chronic sniffling is caused by two completely different conditions: vasomotor rhinitis and allergies.

Vasomotor Rhinitis

I recall an older patient describing how, every time he leaned over a bowl of soup, his nose would run like a faucet. He was concerned that the constant dripping of watery nasal secretions into his broth was costing him lots of chicks/hens. He had tried snorting decongestants, antihistamines, and steroid sprays, all to no avail. But his condition was caused by a short in the wiring of the nasal autonomic nervous system. Welcome to vasomotor rhinitis. Found usually in the older population, this nostril Niagara has nothing to do with allergies. Rather, it is stimulated by changes in temperature, alcohol, and exposure to certain odors and chemicals, including perfumes and newsprint. In fact, if you have vasomotor rhinitis and are reading this book you could well be dripping onto this page, so STOP IT RIGHT NOW! Go and get some Atrovent nasal spray. It works.

Allergies

Another intriguing sign I recall seeing one spring was outside a roadside fruit stand. It read CLOSED FOR THE SEASON, THE REASON IS SNEEZIN'. Allergy sufferers (some 15 per cent of the population) are responsible for more than 2 per cent of all visits to doctor's offices and close to 3 billion dollars a year in medication. Unlike vasomotor rhinitis, allergic rhinitis involves itchiness of the eyes, nose, and roof of the mouth. Usually it is seasonal, but in an unlucky few, it can be perennial, depending on what the allergens are. Common persistent allergic symptoms may necessitate using a Dacron pillow, filtering out house dust, and chucking the cat (which is always fun anyways). If house dust is the culprit, then a humidifier can reduce the amount of dust flying around. If molds are the cause, then a dehumidifier will help.

There is often a family predisposition to allergies. Mornings in some homes are a stereophonic symphony of sneezing. *"Daddy sneezes bass, momma sniffs tenor, and me and little brother drip right in."* Treatment includes the extremely safe nasal steroid sprays, membrane stabilizers, and of course, antihistamines, best taken at night. Those who continue to suffer can go to the increasingly popular desensitization shots. These are usually given weekly for a few months and then tapered to monthly injections. And if you do have to undergo these weekly shots, remember... No Sniveling!

SNORE NO MORE

Usually, I write while perched on a chair at a desk that's covered with so much high-tech equipment that I'm hesitant to push the wrong button for fear of launching cruise missiles into East Kil-gashtania. The beeps and whirls of my IBM are interrupted only by an occasional snore from trusty ol' Murph the hound, who wakes himself up with a loud snort and then glares at me as if I'm to blame.

But today I scribble on a napkin while sitting on a lonely stool in the Goatsucker Saloon, in the middle of the Sonoran Desert of Arizona. The Sonoran Desert prides itself on being named the most beautiful desert on Earth, which may be akin to being the sharpest of the Three Stooges. Much to the chagrin of the Gobi and the Sahara, there actually exist signs stating, "Welcome to the Sonoran Desert, the most beautiful desert in the world." The inhabitants of this desert are elated about this honor. The coyotes are yipping, the lizards are lounging, and the cactus is looking sharp. Sidewinders are beside themselves with excitement. Roadrunners are just running down the road; it's their idea of having fun.

My wife, however, reminds me that the snorin' desert is an action verb, one that describes her leaving the bed as quick as a jackrabbit when I begin my impersonation of a jackhammer in my sleep (a jackass when awake). "Yer a-snorin' agin, so I'm a-desertin' ya till ya git it fixed." How can you tell if you belong in the snorin' desert? You may be one of the 37 million habitual snorers who wake in the morning to find shredded pieces of the bedroom curtain embedded in the back of your throat or large cracks forming in the ceiling above your side of the bed. Perhaps you awake to your near-deaf wife advising you that a crowd of seismologists have congregated on the driveway, searching for an epicenter.

The Colorado River helps maintain life in the Sonoran. The saguaro cactus, to my surprise, grows only in the Sonoran Desert (because of the river). It grows in no other desert in the world. Where the river is wide, the water meanders along peacefully, the silence broken only by an occasional scorpion sneeze. When the river hits a narrow canyon it changes into a raging gorge that is so noisy you can't hear yourself burp. This also explains why we snore. When the back of our throat is wide open, air peacefully flows through. When the throat is narrowed, the air, scurrying past redundant tissue and tongue, makes a loud snore.

So How Can You Snore No More?

1. Lie on your side. When you lie on your back, your tongue falls into the back of your throat, obstructing the flow of air. The old tennis-ball-in-the-back-pocket trick will either keep you on your side or else leave the word "Spalding" branded on your buttock.
2. Discontinue alcohol consumption. It makes everything go floppy and blocks airflow.
3. Lose weight.
4. Consider a dental retainer that thrusts the jaw forward, opening up the back of the throat. But keep in mind that in addition to making you look like Robocop with braces, these devices are expensive and can lead to jaw problems.
5. Look into LAUP (laser-assisted uvulopalatoplasty), the mainstay of treatment. A laser is used to cut out the offending tissue in the back of your throat, the soft palate, and the uvula (that wormlike dangler in the back of your throat that flaps about like crazy when you snore). This is the most common method for definitive snoring treatment and is overwhelmingly recommended by doctors who happen to own lasers. LAUP usually takes only one treatment. It does, however, cause a significant amount of discomfort for the first week or so after treatment, and pain medication is required.
6. Try somnoplasty, a new method that involves firing radio waves into the back of the throat and requires two to three applications to eradicate the snoring apparatus. The radio waves coagulate the tissue in the back of the throat, causing it to contract. No actual cutting of tissue occurs; subsequently, there is no pain. As an added bonus, the FM stations come in really clear.

COMMON SENSE

My grandfather's name was Dah. His real name, I'm told, was George, but to his grandkids he was good ol' Dah. As a wee lad I would spend hours sitting on Dah's lap, watching the oft-resurrected Wile E. Coyote rocket through another Acme disaster, while the burning embers from ol' Dah's cigar would fall into his snowy white chest hair or directly onto my cornea. Finally he would say, "David, you're fifteen years old. Get off my lap and give me back the cigar." I loved ol' Dah, and when he passed away it was for me a cruel joke.

Thirty years after his passing, I received an unexpected phone call.

"Hi, my name is Bugsy, and I fought alongside your grandfather George in Italy."

"You knew Dah?" I exclaimed, thrilled at being reminded of my childhood pal. As Bugsy went on to relate some of Dah's legendary military feats, which usually featured greased pigs, five aces, or stolen jeeps, I began to notice a strange odor at my desk, stranger than normal. I glared at the dog, who glared back with a stupid yet innocent grin on his mug, but it wasn't him.

Suddenly this strange yet familiar smell twanged the memory cells of my brain. It was Dah's cigar. So clearly could I smell that smoke that I had to look around the room twice to ensure that no such cigar was smoldering. Smelling a man dead thirty years may seem a tad Beetlejuicy and perverse, but in the part of my mind responsible for smell, he was very much fresh and alive. Such is the power of the sense of smell.

"DOC, I DON'T smell too good."

"Well, Bloggins, I've got a cold, so I really didn't notice..."

"No, I mean I can't smell anything anymore. On occasion it's a blessing, but for the most part, it drives me nuts. And when I eat, I can't tell if I'm eating the pizza or the cardboard box. I'm about as interested in food as I am in vacationing in Chechnya.

Worse yet, it's really getting me down. Life seems to have lost its zest for me lately."

AT THE ROOF of our nose, in a happy little bone called the cribriform plate, sits the olfactory bulb, an organ lined with kazillions of glomeruli. These amazing smell cells can detect, differentiate, and process ten thousand different smells. While taste buds have four basic tastes—salty, sweet, sour, and Black Forest cake—the sense of smell allows us to identify exactly what we have just placed in our mouth. When an odor, nice or nasty, wafts into our nostrils past assorted hairs, chalk, and fingernails, the glomeruli process the odor, pack up the information, and fire it along the olfactory nerve to some place in the brain right next to the "It-Wasn't-Me!" denial center.

Anosmia refers to the complete loss of smell. The commonest causes of anosmia include:

· sinus disease (either allergic or infectious),
· upper respiratory infections, which is why normally evil-tasting beasts such as Buckley's or Fisherman's Friend can actually be tolerated when we have a cold,
· head trauma, which can disrupt the cribriform plate in the nose.

Half of those over age sixty have some olfactory dysfunction not necessarily related to any disease, unless you term aging a disease. As we age, our sense of smell joins the vision and hearing in a gradual decline. Rather than young vibrant cells working hard in the olfactory center, old factory workers now go on strike. Smoking helps to wear down the old factory workers even further. A lack of smell is associated with increased depression and a lower quality of life. Thus it can be concluded that smoking contributes to depression.

Astonishingly, loss of smell can also be an early marker for certain neurodegenerative diseases such as Parkinson's, Alzheimer's, and even multiple sclerosis. In fact, anosmia may be the first symptom to signal the onset of these diseases.

As for you, Dah, thanks for knocking some "sense" back into me. Smell ya later.

COLLECTION AGENCY

I collect license plates. A peculiar hobby to be sure, but I find it to be relatively inexpensive, spine-tingling fun. Requirements: one flashlight, one screwdriver, two good sneakers, one police scanner. I have been fascinated with plates since the day my mother dragged me by the hand through a busy Sears parking lot and I came across a Hawaiian license plate. Certain things make a lifelong impression when you're seventeen. And so to this day, to identify an exotic plate ahead of me on the road, I will hit the high beams and zip my Plymouth Fury to within a few electrons of the rear license of an alarmed Oregonian or Wyomingite. I get right excited when an Alaska, Rhode Island, or Newfoundland plate crosses my path. It's also a practical hobby. Having a collection of plates not only makes for great pranks ("I'm sure we parked over here somewhere, Mildred"), but it also gives me something to aim my .22 at, besides stoplights, taillights, and Fifi next door.

Most people collect something, even if it's just plaque between their teeth or lint between their toes. My brake-pedal-challenged son collects speeding tickets. I believe he's close to getting an entire set with police signatures from all the precincts. A urologist friend collects large or odd-shaped kidney stones and relishes showing off the various fascinating shapes and sizes of stones he removed from patients, all the while relating the pain this poor patient or the other must have experienced. One desperate collector paid ten thousand dollars for a piece of gum chewed by a baseball player, no doubt to add to his collection of pre-chewed celebrity food.

Some poor souls collect diseases. "Why is it, doctor, that I seem to collect every bug in the book? While my wife couldn't catch a cold if she hitchhiked through Greenland naked, I collect a virus every time someone in another time zone sneezes in my direction."

Why is it that some people constantly get ill, while others have the constitution of a rock? Are their immune systems weak? Can "weak" immune systems be enhanced?

I don't know. So I asked an immunologist/pitching wedge specialist.

"Our immune system's ability to be fully operational can certainly be affected by lack of sleep, jet lag, nutritional status, age, underlying diseases, physical activity, stress and even personal hygiene," he said. "Oddly enough, we may be too rigorous about hygiene in our society. A fascinating theory known as the Hygiene Hypothesis claims that we might actually be living in too clean an environment. Kids who are exposed to a lot of viruses (i.e., a lot of other kids) at an earlier time in their life seem to have fewer problems with allergies, asthma, and other immune-related problems when they get older. Those who have never been ill as a kid are known as 'naive,' meaning that they might not have developed immunity to many common bugs and you can easily yank them an atomic wedgie. Put them into school, a virtual cesspool of viruses, and they become a collection agency for every bug in the school."

How to Enhance Your Immune System

1. Be active. A study out of the University of South Carolina showed that physically active people had 23 per cent fewer colds than couch potatoes. In the fall, when about 40 per cent of all colds occur, the risk reduction was a whooping 32 per cent less in the active group: nothing to sniff at.

2. Breastfeed. (Must be age appropriate.) Breastfed babes have their immune system charged early and well.

3. Immunize, immunize, location. The immune system has a terrific memory. Each time it encounters a virus it has seen before,

it acts faster and faster to destroy the invader. Billions and billions of T cells (the mainstay of the immune system) patrol the body and scan over every jot and tittle to see if it belongs in our body or if it is a foreigner that needs to be destroyed. Vaccines prime this immune system. The flu shot boosts the immune system so well that those who get them suffer fewer colds and flu.

4. Reimmunize. As we age, our immune system's memory develops Alzheimer's, meaning that our T cells forget why they opened the fridge. As the memory of foreign invaders fades we need to revisit booster shots in the older population.

5. Get your immunonutrients. Evidence is mounting that our immune response during an infection might be improved by increasing our collection of certain nutrients, including glutamine, arginine, and long-chain polyunsaturated fatty acids, none of which need to be . . . pre-chewed.

ROCK ON

Recently I slud into seductive Sedona, Arizona, the happy, hippie home of mystical magical mountains and ridiculously red rocks. A town where inhabitants proudly proclaim to be "diagonally parked in a parallel universe." Or, as an ol' timer explained as he looked me over suspiciously, "Yep, since the rocks supposedly got magical powers, we got every fruitcake in the pantry coming here now." Enclosing this desert town are fascinating rock formations nicknamed by the locals after who or what they resemble. These rocks are blessed with mystical powers that apparently can heal hernias, soothe snakebites, cure consumption, remedy rheumatizz, treat tremors, and purge pinworms, all while magically levitating twenty-dollar bills out of tourist wallets. Nature has formed these monolithic monsters into Merry-Go-Round Rock, Coffeepot Rock, Snoopy Rock, and Devil's Bridge.

Nature also forms rocks in our bodies. We name them after what organ seems to be closest to them. But unlike Sedona, our rocks are not cures, but rather corrupters. Typically, human stones obstruct the free flow of fluids, leading to swelling and severe pain.

Gallstones
Thirty million North Americans carry gallstones in their gall-bladders. Collectively, that actually adds up to a whopping forty tons of rock, also known as a Mama Cass/Meatloaf duet. Another one million of you will be diagnosed with cholelithia-sis (gallstones) this year. Half will have them removed surgically. Usually these stones, 75 per cent of which are cholesterol stones, laze around the bottom of the gallbladder and never venture out on tour. If they do get squeezed out into the bile duct, then all heck breaks loose. Sometimes they will slide back into the gall bag, but often they will stay put, creating major pain just under the right breast (which, in my granny, may be confused with knee pain). Ninety per cent of the time, surgery is the method of choice for removal of impacted gallstones. Only a small per-centage fit the criteria for lithotripsy, whereby ultrasonic waves shatter the stone into small bits.

Sialolithiasis, or stones of the saliva glands
Open your mouth and look under your tongue at the floor of your mouth. Remove parsley. See those two disgusting clammy-looking fellas peeking up? Those are Wharton's ducts, named after the salivalologist who discovered them, Dr. Ducts. Can't find them? Then place a lemon in your mouth and watch what happens. Stones can form in this duct too, getting stuck and causing pain and swelling under the chin and in the neck.

Prostatic calculi
As if the prostate doesn't have enough problems, small stones form in the prostates of 75 per cent of middle-aged men and 100 per cent of elderly men. Though usually not symptomatic, these stones can get infected and remain a source of chronic bladder infections.

Fecalith

Concretion of the feces can occur so that a piece of hardened feces becomes a nasty round stone (rabbit rocks) and gets jammed somewhere in the intestinal system. Fecaliths are the commonest cause of appendicitis as well as diverticulitis (which is often described as appendicitis on the left side of the abdomen).

Kidney stones·

Last but not least are the horrifically painful kidney stones.

Kidney stones, also known as uroliths, hurt; they really hurt. Unlike appendicitis, where the patient tends to lie quite still wanting no one to touch them, the kidney stoner cannot seem to find a comfortable position, tossing to and fro during the colicky attacks.

Depending on the size and location of the stone, hours or even weeks may pass before it does. Pain killers and anti-inflammatory suppositories are used until the stone passes. The patient is also given a urine strainer in order to try and catch the stone so it can be analyzed. Please dispose of these strainers carefully, especially when at the office. ("Bloggins, the coffee has a bit of an aftertaste since I used that new filter you brought in. Got any breath mints?")

Should you catch the stone, it will be sent off to a kidney stonologist who, 80 per cent of the time, will report that the stone is composed of calcium oxalate. Ten per cent will have the uric acid stones of gout.

Sometimes the stone does not pass at all. Lithotripsy is a process whereby the stone is shattered while still in the urinary tract. Ultrasonic shock waves or even laser blasters can be used to reduce the stone to stubble. It's a urologist's arcade.

Thirty per cent of those with one attack will have a subsequent attack within a year. To avoid stone formations, they are advised to:

· Increase fluid intake to more than four pints per day. Oddly enough, most stone formers have an abhorrence of drinking fluids.

- Limit protein intake to about two grams per pound of your weight per day. Too much protein attracts more calcium into your blood and urine and, much to your un-satisfaction, you will form rolling stones. Speaking of Keith Richards, drug addicts with "high" aspirations like to use the kidney-stone ruse. They arrive in the ER with allergies to everything but narcotics, toss a little blood into their urine sample, then writhe about in pain.
- Avoid salt. Like protein, salt causes more calcium to build up in the kidneys.
- Do not restrict your calcium intake. As odd as this may sound, decreasing your intake of calcium may actually increase your absorption of oxalates, and it is the oxalate intake that tends to be the problem. Oxalates are found in chocolate, peanuts, and tea.

One million North Americans will get kidney stones this year. Dehydration is one of the commonest causes of these hot rocks, which is why it is important to avoid hot, rocky, seductive desert towns. Otherwise... rock on, Sedona.

SMACKULAR DEGENERATES

I caught the Perseid meteor showers last summer, or at least I watched them, or at least I tried to. August's celestial showcase, performed on the northeast stage of heaven's amphitheatre, is an exercise in aggravation to many of us who would actually like to see this shooting-star spectacle. As I lay flat on the long grass with my young son, dew, dirt, and various vile invertebrates violating my ear canals, he would point quickly: "See that one, Dad?"

Yeah! Well, almost. More like "not really, but I think I just got bit." By the time I directed my gaze to the streak that I thought I saw in my peripheral vision, the show was over. Traveling at forty miles per second, or just slightly slower than my eldest son's pickup truck and pickup lines, streaking stars are not always easy for these old degenerate eyes to track.

To 10 per cent of those older than sixty-five years of age and to 30 per cent of those beyond seventy-five, peripheral vision may be all that actually works anymore. The macula, a small area in the back of the eye (retina) responsible for central vision, can degenerate all too easily. In fact, far too many of the Edsel/ Eisenhower/Elvis generation are now in a general state of degeneration. Bones, joints, memory, muscles, hearing, vision, and other organs of various size and function all begin to shrivel as we begin our free fall into the world of senescence, one we all too often have not prepared properly for. Even the invincible Britney generation needs to prepare now to eventually join the degenerate generation.

Macular degeneration (MD, also known as "smackular" degeneration given the many times that foreheads become intimately acquainted with telephone poles, baseballs, and oncoming wheelchairs) causes loss of "straight ahead" vision in both eyes. This makes simple tasks like reading, driving, and ogling intolerable.

The macula can be wrecked in two ways. It may be invaded by a horde of leaky blood vessels that destroy the macula, the so-called "wet" macular degeneration. Or, in "dry" degeneration, which accounts for 90 per cent of MD, the macula may just start to shrivel and break down, slowly causing vision to blur and dark patches to emerge in the middle of a sentence. For example, if a newspaper's health column were juxtaposed with a gardening column, there might be large gaps in the center of your vision, leading to sentences such as:

· to prevent nose bleeds: don't pick too early and always check for beetles

· the eye surgeon might: use a large-toothed 22-horsepower rototiller

· if not circumcised, a boy might discover: an aggressive Venus flytrap

· side effects include: spreading a large amount of manure and worms about the bed

Wet MD causes a more profound blindness and is responsible for 80 per cent of legally blind eyes. But if it is caught early, thermal laser treatment and hours of fervent prayer may be able to slow wet destruction of the macula. Macular degeneration may not always render its victims blind, but it might reduce them from fully sighted to partially sighted. Still, loss of central vision can lead to loss of driver's license, loss of autonomy, and loss of joie de vivre. Although sun exposure, high blood pressure, and lack of zinc have all been named as possible causes of MD, the only proven risk factor is our old friend smoking. After smoke gets in your eyes, don't it make your brown eyes blue.

According to eye specialists (MD MDs), it is recommended that you:

· not ignore any blind spots, blurriness, wavy lines, or decrease in color vision. See a doctor who will test your central vision with an Amsler grid. You can easily find an Amsler grid on the Internet and test your central vision at home.

· have an eye exam (both eyes) every two years if you are over age sixty-five, every year if you smoke.

· not sit in the foul-ball section as you begin to age.

But most importantly, remember that you will invariably go blind unless you ask your doctor to: clip your begonias each fall.

TERMINAL ILLNESS

My office staff, having never served in government, seldom misses work because of illness. But every April 1, the most wonderful time of the year in the hap-happiest place on Earth, they seem to collectively get ill: "Sorry, but I have pints of purulent pus pouring out of my pancreas. I have to go see a real doctor." "Can't come in today, my dog's fleas are expecting anytime now."

Initially I suspected they were simply at home celebrating this joyous of all days, but then it dawned on me that perhaps sliding off toilet seats, being blamed for sounds emitted by electronic whoopee cushions, and other sophisticated pranks customary to my office was finally getting to them.

. So last year I snuck in early, went to their computer terminals, popped a few tabs off their keyboards, and exchanged them with each other. The M and the N changed positions, as did the P and the L and even the ! and the $. Little did I realize the havoc this would wreak; Elana couldn't access her password, Michelle was billing $17,000 for Bill Bloggins' pregnancy test, and a flustered Betty was unable to move the jack of hearts. They became frantic and unsure of what evil was causing this terminal illness. I was in April Fool's heaven.

In addition to a malfunctioning computer driving its victims to extremes of mental anguish, several other terminal illnesses are generated by the keyboard, the monitor, the mouse, and even by the laptop.

- Eye troubles. A recent study has related heavy computer use with visual field abnormalities, refractive errors, and glaucoma. Visual field defects means having blind spots in the normal visual field. Think umpires. A refractive error is an inability to see clearly without corrective lenses. Think refs. Glaucoma refers to a pressure buildup in the eyeball itself that affects vision and makes halos around bright lights. Think Dr. Dave.
- Infertility in men. The reason that the male testicles are not normally tucked up, say, into the Adam's apple (polar bear swims excluded) is that sperm production requires a temperature lower than that of the body's core. From the "Excuse-me-but-you're-going-to-stick-that-temperature-gauge-where?" file comes a study that indicates that sixty minutes of a laptop sitting on the lap top raises scrotal temperature almost three degrees. Even if the laptop was not turned on (perhaps I should rephrase that), there was

a two-degree rise. "Don't worry about the birth control pill, dear, I've taken my laptop today."

· Tennis elbow belongs to a group of injuries known as cumulative trauma disorders (CTD). Also called repetitive strain injury, CTDs result from repetitive exertion of a tendon, muscle, joint, or even bone. Excessive typing can ruin the tendons responsible for moving the wrist/hand/fingers up and down. When discomfort is felt up in the elbow or upper forearm, see a doctor before the strain, sprain, or pain becomes debilitating. CTD (can't type, dammit) can become so severe over time that even holding a glass becomes a chore. This condition is one of the fastest-growing injuries in the workplace. Even with proper ergonomics of the keyboard, monitor, mouse, chair, and desk, too much time spent on a keyboard may mean too much time spent in physiotherapy.

· Way back when I went to college, the most common illnesses were smallpox, bubonic plague, and consumption. Now depression and non-activity exhaustion, which go hand in hand with heavy computer use, are the most prevalent illnesses on most college campuses. Students are still working on consumption.

· Muscle contraction headaches—so-called tension headaches— result from the neck and back stiffening up while perched at a computer all day. In addition, migraines and even seizures can be triggered by the flickering of a computer screen. "Monitor eye" is a type of eyestrain that causes fuzzy vision and headaches. But the vurst type of headacke is caused by tryink to fiqure out who monceyed arount with your conpuder on Aqril $st. I wist you the pest of thus joyouz zeazon;.

MORTON HEARS A BOO-HOO

Don't look now, but your body is being brutally damaged by something you're wearing. Tongue stud? Tight Fruit of the Looms? Barry Manilow T-shirt? Sure, but even worse are your loafers, pumps, and stilettos.

A study conducted in China several years ago compared the relationship between footwear and foot problems. It concluded that umpteen billion Chinese who did not wear shoes seldom had foot problems, while the other umpteen billion who wore shoes suffered bunions, ingrown toenails, corns, and painful swollen nerves called "neuromas."

A neuroma of the foot, known as a Morton's neuroma, is a painful pain or a numbing numbness involving the ball of the foot and the third and fourth toes (sometimes the second and third toes). When the nerve that meanders through the foot en route to the toes gets squished between the bones of the foot, a neuroma develops. This pressure irritates the nerve and, much like an oyster's irritated sand pebble turns into a lovely lump known as a pearl, the nerve turns into a nasty lump known as a neuroma. Eighty per cent of those with Morton's neuroma are female, a result of high heels and tight toe boxes that incarcerate their dainty wee hooves.

The foot nerves can also be irritated by trauma, as when a wheelie-poppin' teenage terror operating the forklift at Costco screams around a corner and runs over your foot. Literally gets on your "nerves."

Treatment of this condition requires changing to footwear with a more spacious toe box. Adding the highly popular orthotics (shoe inserts) is highly effective at battling most of the archenemies of several foot problems. Since the foot bone is connected to the leg bone, these same orthotics can correct ankle, knee, hip, and back problems, and even alleviate some forms of headache. If orthotics fail, the next step of treatment involves a painful cortisone shot directly into the neuroma.

I have decided to feet-ure neuromas in this book because... well, I have one myself. Yes, my name is Dave and... I am a Morton's neuromic.

Though my condition has improved since giving up the high heels (just kidding—to be honest, my very rugged manly hockey skates squeeze my foot), the pain was bad enough for me to undergo the cortisone procedure.

I went to my colleague and trusted surgeon, Dr. "Butch" Butcher.

First, the necessary acknowledgments.

"Doctor."

"Doctor."

"Doctor, I need a Morton's neuroma doctored."

"Well, doctor, we'll doctor that right up."

"Thank you, I trust you are still trusted as in the intro I gave you six lines ago."

"Trust me, doctor, I'm a trusted doctor."

Why do doctors make such lousy patients? Is it because they can visualize the worst possible scenarios? In medical school, we were all convinced we had whatever disease we happened to be studying that week. We checked ourselves for lymphoma lumps, testicular tumors, and syphilis sores. Prostate cancer week was not a pretty sight on our campus. During obstetrics, we devoured pistachio dill pickle ice cream and our feet swelled.

So, do I handle this procedure of having a needle jammed between my toes like a man or like a doctor? I tell myself that, as a doctor, I can visualize the afferent nerve conduction pathways as the plexus of nerve cells succumb to the membrane channel-blocking ion-exchange proton-pump inhibitor. As a man, I search the room desperately for Mr. Wiggles, my stuffed glow-worm, because this is going to be one big owwie.

A week later, at home licking my wounds (figuratively speaking), I ponder my new resolution to improve my foot health. Though I'm now asked to leave restaurants, my pew at church is deserted, and patients peer at me suspiciously, I think going barefoot has been therapeutic. It really is the best thing you can do for your feet.

Trust me, I'm a doctor.

FUNGUS AMONG US

1. The commonest complaint heard in a doctor's office is (choose one):
   a. "My back hurts."
   b. "I've got a rash."
   c. "I have an acutely inflamed neuralgia involving the second branch of the fifth cranial nerve."
   d. "Doctor, you're standing on my broken foot."
   The correct answer is b.

2. Which irritating skin condition is most common?
   a. measles rash
   b. toenail fungus
   c. heat rash
   d. a rash of irrational politicians making rash decisions (putting us all on rations)
   The correct answer is b (although politicians and toenail fungus are technically similar).

3. Which one does not belong?
   a. athlete's foot
   b. skier's thumb
   c. jock itch
   d. ringworm
   e. toenail fungus
   The correct answer is b, as a, c, d, and e are all caused by the very same type of skin fungus.

4. What percentage of the population has toenail fungus?
   a. .007 per cent
   b. c and e
   c. 5 per cent of those over age fifty-five
   d. 210 per cent
   e. 2 per cent

The correct answer is b. In addition, more than 50 per cent of the population may have a fungal skin infection at any given time.

If you answered all four questions correctly, then you
a. are a doctor of great repute
b. realize that most doctors passed exams by always answering b
c. cheated
d. have terminal toenail fungus

ONYCHOMYCOSIS (worth big points in Scrabble) is the term for nails that turn yellowish, flaky, cracked, and as thick as Mike Tyson's cranium. Though one may feel that treating toenail fungus is purely a cosmetic thing, the goalie from my hockey team, Don, recently proved that this disease stretches beyond mere vanity. He approached me with a concern that he might have toenail fungus. I had him remove his skates and the Miss Clairol Ruby Red nail polish and sure enough... a fifty-seven-point Scrabble score. The next week I noted that Don had become withdrawn and introverted, and had resorted to a darker maroon polish. He looked at me between tears and sobbed, "Why me?" Indeed, I was witnessing the heartbreak of onychomycosis.

Not realizing that I was pushing him to the brink, I pointed out several round red marks on his torso that he had mistaken for missed pucks and revealed, "Donnie, you've also got ringworm." As the rest of the team made a mad dash for the door at the mention of "worms," I called them back and explained that Donnie's puck marks were not really worms at all, as "ringworm" is a misnomer. The red raised perimeter of these lesions makes it look as though a worm has burrowed in a circle under the skin. I explained that this was simply a nasty, highly infectious, superficial skin fungus, at which time the team made a mad dash for the door.

Worms are pretty bummed out about the bad PR. All they want from life is to wake up earlier than early birds, soak at the bottom of a tub of tequila, and go fishing. Same is true of athletes, who are perturbed by such terms as athlete's foot, jock itch, etc. All they want from life is to wake up late, soak in a tub of tequila, and fish around in their jocks on national TV.

I had Donnie use some vaginal yeast cream and the puck marks disappeared, along with his PMS. He took an antifungal pill, and four months later the toenail fungus disappeared. Should Donnie read this, I, too, might disappear. Fortunately for me, there are no cartoons in this book.

WHAT A FLAKE

For more than two thousand years, myth information about bloodletting had wealthy Europeans attempting to rid the body of "excess blood caused by excess food." The favored method for bloodletting—prior to leeches, the NHL, and tax collectors—was a bimonthly trip to the barber. Barbaric barbers from the Barbary Coast to Barbados had the snappiest razors for slicing open arms, legs, feet, the rump, and even the tongue. These barbershops were marked with a white and red pole, signifying a white bandage wrapped around a bloody arm.

My own barberette is a salty, insulting Maritimer named Angie, who engages in a constant barrage of barbs while I sit handcuffed to the red chair of death. Any attempt at a retort to this evil connoisseur of coifs is met with a stiff slap upside the head and a threat to resume the ancient barber right of ear slicing. This is her room and she is in charge. The insults come hard and low, from the moment she slaps the leg irons on my shins right up until the ambulance arrives.

Her banter, no doubt meant to distract me from my hemorrhagic state:

"Man, your hair is getting gray; oh, wait, it's not gray, just this salt mine of dandruff you have everywhere other than this huge mother-of-a-crater of a bald spot, but hey, don't worry about your

monk patch, 'cause you're not really losing your hair, it's just relo-
cated to your nose, ears, and eyebrows." With that she produces
some witchy whirling weed-whacking wand and rams it up my
nose, into my ears, and across my brows. "Man, your head is as
flaky as Michael Jackson's. Not fair of you to make skiers and
snowboarders salivate every time you shake your head."

"Now wait one minute, Angie, you. . ."

SLAP. NICK.

Dandruff, plaguing a whopping 50 per cent of North Americans, can range from mild flaking to full-scale (sorry) scalp
psoriasis. The human scalp normally sheds itself quietly over a
twenty-eight-day period, unless you've inadvertently married
Henry VIII. Fine particles of dead skin fall off without ever being
seen. Those with dandruff, however, shed their scales in a more
accelerated seven to twenty-one days. These dead skin cells are
shed so quickly that they clump together, creating flakes. While
genetics and climate play a role in how fast the skin turns over,
a fancy wee fungus named *Malassezia furfur* (need a unique
name for the next kid?) often sets up shop in the scalp, triggering
a hyperproliferation of the scalp's epidermis. Other factors that
cause the scalp to be drier and flakier include conditions that
usually make skin drier in general:

- Weather. October to March is dandruff season, but a hot summer
  sun can also dry out the skin.
- Blow-dryers. By creating a desert sirocco on your head, you create
  dunes of dry skin.
- Wool hats.
- Picking and scratching.
- Stress. Too much stress can create dandruff! Executive Scalp Syndrome describes excessive dandruff in young, stressed-out execu-
  tives. Yes, these guys are head and shoulders above the rest of us.
- Hair care products: colorants, fragrances, gels, mousse, mice,
  moose.

Treatment of dandruff is varied. Zinc pyrithione (Head & Shoulders) addresses the fast-shedding skin, while Nizoral and selenium sulfide (Selsun) go after poor *Malassezia*. A really inflamed scalp may need a steroid lotion. For really prolific dandruff the tar shampoos may be needed, though your head may give off a pong like a highway in a heat wave. Does not go well with your feather boa. I find that when I'm in doubt of which product to use to cure my scalp problem, I consult the nearest medical source: the ambulance driver.

BLEEBIE HEEBIE JEEBIES

If you could be a doctor for a day, what kind of doctor would you be? Surgeon, GP, cardiologist, George Clooney, Dr. Hook? What if you had to decide on the type of doctoring you would malpractice every day for the rest of your life? Such a decision is one that all medical students must make as they edge closer to actually obtaining their MD (Master of Deception). Those who don't mind spending a total of forty-seven seconds per week with their family choose surgery. Those who feel sleep is a waste of time go into obstetrics. Those who enjoy working for $1.67/hour become GPs. But the smart ones become dermatologists, the rare breed of doctor who enjoys a nine-to-five lifestyle; big, beautiful bodacious sports cars, and pustular acne. A ruptured pimple, even at 3:00 AM on the night before an audition for, say, *Survivor Winnipeg*, seldom carries the same degree of urgency as a ruptured aorta. Extricating excess lint from a belly button is seldom as critical as extricating a harpoon from a carotid. A raging wart isn't associated with the same fear as a raging granny.

Yet abdominal pain and rashes tend to be the toughest problems for most GPs to solve. A patient can often be panic-stricken about an intense rash, one that I might not recognize. Adding, "Wow, I have never seen one that color before, at least not on a live patient!" tends to convert their panic into frenzied terror.

So on occasion, I call up a helpful dermatologist, the nicest of all specialists (something to do with eight hours' sleep), who calmly solves the carcass conundrum. They are expert rashologists, toenailologists, and bleebieologists. Knowing about a few common bleebies may save you unnecessary panic. So, while I close my eyes, you should remove all of your clothes, get out a mirror, and check for:

Seborrheic Keratoses
Often mistaken for moles or warts, sks are, next to moles, the most common skin lesion. Seen in the aging population (i.e., those whose actions creak louder than their words), sks are found primarily on the trunk, back, face, and hands. They have a tan color and a stuck-on appearance, meaning that they are part of the outer layer of skin (epidermis). Those with several sks look as though they have rolled naked in a field of light brown gum. An sk might be a large, thick, hard wad of gum or a small, thin piece. And, like gum, sks can virtually be scraped off the skin with a dinner knife and flicked across the table for a little dining fun. If you consider scraping them off to be uncouth, then try gnawing them off with your teeth (for those hard-to-reach sks, remove dentures and start chomping). Should you be blessed with a more refined upbringing than my own, see a doctor, who will freeze them off with liquid nitrogen or scrape them off with a cheese grater.

Skin Tags
These do not turn into cancer. Fifty per cent of these wee cauliflowers are found in the armpits, 35 per cent on the neck, and the rest in the groin. Tags typically hang on a stalk like a floppy little mushroom and get caught on clothing or necklaces, camera straps, purse straps, Right Guard, backpacks, fingernails, the cat, ponytails, Ban Roll-on, tree branches, zz Top, mink stoles, and the like. A good-sized tag can tear into Grandma's pearl necklace like it was Silly String. Have those tags snipped or frozen off.

Basal Cell Cancer

A dermatologist once took me for a stroll and pointed out numerous people walking about sporting BCCs on their mugs. This most common of the skin cancers has a pearly white border and occurs only in the white population. BCCs are sun-sensitive tumors, 85 per cent of which occur on the face, 30 per cent on the nose alone. Not an aggressive cancer, this basal cell cancer does not metastasize but invades the skin, eating away at the nose like Michael Jackson's plastic surgeon.

BUT IF YOU'RE at all in doubt about a bleebie or any mysterious lump or bump, be sure to have it checked out by a professional such as George Clooney. He can be reached at www.drdavelookalike.com.

WART WARS

I feinted left, but he was too quick and caught me with a crisp jab. As my head snapped back, I glimpsed an opening and landed a twisting uppercut to his chin. He reeled, and I followed with a sweeping right hook to the temple that buckled his knees. He backpedaled to a corner, so I moved in. Countering, he connected with a devastating combination jab/hook that momentarily stunned me. I fell back. But seven years of college hockey (I had a long college career) had trained me well. I answered with a stiff jab to his flaring nostrils, but he answered right back with a kick to my midsection. So I reached for a bottle of liquid nitrogen, grabbed his flailing foot, and worked him hard.

A minute later, it was all over.

"Thanks, doctor, I hope little Mikey wasn't too tough on you. Should we come back next week for another liquid nitrogen treatment of his wart?"

While kids might hate warts, they despise wart treatment and positively loathe wart treaters. To those who feel that the above struggle is not entirely plausible, I should advise you that my PG-13 rating prevents me from including the really vicious portions of the battle that involved teeth, scalpels, and Tonya Harding.

All this fuss over a virus no bigger than a mosquito's zit. Warts are caused by HPV, known as human papilloma virus or more commonly the horrific pimple virus. It enters through a breach in the skin and may take months or even years to incubate. Different types of warts are caused by different varieties of the seventy strains of HPV, including:

· PLANTAR WART: Warts on the feet are a common adolescent concern. Plantar warts begin on the weight-bearing portions of the foot and are so named because as they enlarge, walking feels as though a Planters Peanut is embedded in the foot. Warts are "caught" from public showers or from swapping low-fives with warty friends. What may start as a single wart may multiply into several warts, which may in turn fuse into large plaques that can consume the entire soul of the foot. To treat: pare down the wart until it begins to bleed, then freeze with liquid nitrogen (use the spray only, not a cotton swab); thaw, freeze again, then cross fingers.

· SUBUNGUAL WARTS: Found under and adjacent to the fingernails, these warts are notoriously persistent and painful to treat. Some success is found with 5 per cent imiquimod, a rather expensive cream that is applied after soaking and filing down the wart.

· COMMON WARTS: ten per cent of the general population have warts. Fifty per cent of warts will disappear spontaneously within two years. These warts should be soaked in warm water, pared or pumiced, soaked again, treated with a chemical weapon (acids, cantharidin, podofilm), and then covered with tape or plastic for several days. If all else fails, liquid nitrogen *might* work.

· FLAT WARTS: Small, flat warts are usually found on the top of the hand or on the face. They are easily spread on shaved areas, such as the legs of women and beards of men (or vice versa).

· GENITAL WARTS: Extremely common among sexually active teens; debate continues as to whether condoms protect or not. Though not exactly the same HPV that causes cervical cancer, the presence of genital warts is a red flag for potential cervical cancer. They are tough and painful to treat (physically and emotionally).

SO FRIENDS, parents, countrymen, send us your ears, your downtrodden, and your donations. But hesitate before sending us kids with warts. The pain they incur from our "treatments" induces a fear reflex between patient and doctor. Years later, when they need to see a doctor for something less painful like a ruptured liver or javelin accident, all they can think of is the pain associated with wart treatment from the guy in the white coat and brass knuckles. "Doc, go ahead and wiggle that javelin in there all you like; just don't use your liquid nitrogen."

And now, as my day comes to a close, my nurse informs me, "Doctor, four-year-old Suzy Stallone is here with a plantar, and she looks like she could go five rounds or more." Thwarted again.

MATTERS
(*of the* HEART)
& BRAIN

HEARTFELT SNOW ANGELS

To prepare for hours of freestyle couching during the Winter
Olympics, I decided to get the mood by going skiing. This would
be downhill skiing, as in plop my thermally protected keyster
onto a cushy chair, ride comfortably to the top of a big hill, turn
the pointy end of the skis back toward the restaurant, hang on
to somebody soft, and slide sweetly down the slopes. The only
exercise I ever seem to get, however, is when I go into my kami-
kaze combat tuck just prior to plowing into an unsuspecting ski
school of six-year-olds. I have developed quite a talent for knocking down one key skier, who in turn wipes out the rest of the
hapless class ("Downhill Domino Dave").

But on this particular day, the mountain was cloaked in a
cold, windy, thick January fog. So in keeping with my annual
resolve to experience two new adventures each year, I decided to
go down to the sheltered woods and try my hand at cross-country
skiing. It turns out that cross-country skiing is as similar to downhill skiing as water-skiing is to fishing.

To begin with, the "Nordic" ski lodge was different from
downhill ski lodges. Wishing to begin my adventure with some

nutritional support, I made for the cafeteria. But my order of "fries and root beer" seemed to render the entire bustling lodge of horrified muesli-fed skiers instantly catatonic. "Sir, don't you mean alfalfa and Evian?"

I rented my gear and headed off.

"First time, sir?" asked Hans, as he handed me the poles.

"Why, yes, how did you know?"

"Just a guess," stated the young blond machine, staring at my post-Christmas flabdomen. "Thought you might vont a lesson."

"No way!" I replied indignantly. "I'm a hockey player. I can certainly figure this out." But twenty-seven minutes and several snow angels later, I was one of six students listening to Hans explain the skill of double poling. Among a group of little Helgas and Svetlanas, I was the only student with a name pronounceable by George W. Bush. But the lesson paid off, and I soon kicked away from the class of preschoolers and headed off into the peaceful, pastoral, and picturesque woods. Pausing recumbent in the snow-angel position, I soaked up the Frost poetry (Robert and Jack) scene as puffy, light snowflakes drifted gently between the cedars. The silence was disturbed only by my heartbeat. And what a heartbeat it was! My neck felt like it was hosting a jackhammer convention. My pulse was too fast, and I knew I had to slow it down.

What an amazing organ the heart is. This remarkable pump calculates how fast it must beat in order for our muscles or organs to perform the tasks we demand of them. It then pumps the required amount of oxygen-drenched blood to the necessary muscles. But if we get carried away and demand too much blood, the heart will pound away so fast that it can seize up. Heart muscle, like any other muscle, must be exercised or it becomes less and less efficient over time. Perhaps the reason that the average sixty-five-year-old Swede has a stronger heart than the average thirty-year-old beer-swilling North American is that the Swede has to put these skis on each time he goes out to milk the reindeer.

So how fast is too fast? Charts are available at every gym and pool to help determine a decent target heart rate (THR) and a dangerous one. These are generally calculated on a formula of (220 minus your age) × ¾. Warming up slowly to your THR and staying there for thirty minutes, four times a week is absolutely necessary for good pump maintenance. Obese, hypertensive, sedentary, and older patients who want to avoid pump failure need to see a doctor prior to stressing the heart. Lazy lack of attention to the pump is the leading cause of death in our society.

What kind of condition is your heart in? One way to determine your cardio fitness level is to see how long it takes for your heart to return to its resting pulse after exercise. Measure your pulse rate exactly one minute after stopping. If your heart does not slow down at least thirty beats in the first minute, your ticker is hurtin' and at increased risk for a heart attack. If your heart rate slows down more than fifty beats in the first minute, you are ready for the Olympics. I marvel at the biathletes who ski like fiends with their heart racing away and then pause as they prepare their rifles while their heart rate drops enough for them to steady their aim.

And while normally I can't relish skiing with a rifle strapped to my back, I do wish I had one today as a response to the next Viking who stops to ask me if I'm okay while I'm really busy perfecting my snow angels.

DECREASE DA GREASE

Have you, as a patient, ever been concerned that maybe, just maybe, your doctor is not a real doctor? Certainly most of my patients have. Next time, perhaps, just before your "doctor" asks you to perform some undignified neurological test like sticking out your tongue and wiggling your ears while dancing the Macarena, test him out. Mention the word "Framingham." If he responds with a blank stare, you'd best make a run for it—he is a fraud, an herbologist, or possibly 007 in disguise. If he recoils in fear to a distant corner of the room, adopts the fetal position, and starts rocking back and forth, then you are in good hands. He is a real doctor having med school flashbacks. A doctor may not remember which of the kids in the waiting room are his own; he may forget the name of the thingamajiggy in the back of your throat or what vital organ he just removed from your body; but he'll always remember the word Framingham, heard in every second class in medical school.

In 1948, the small town of Framingham, Massachusetts, was selected to undergo the most important study in the history of medicine: the "Framingham Study." Five thousand adults from this town were poked, prodded, and probed over their entire lifetime in order to determine the risk factors for what was becoming a common condition, heart disease. In 1971 another 5,000 Framinghamites, offspring of the original five thou, were also recruited into this ongoing study. Much of what we know today about cardiovascular disease stems from this town. We've learned, among many other things, that the big three risk factors for cardiac disease are smoking, high blood pressure, and high cholesterol.

Q. So are you saying that cholesterol is bad then, doctor?
A. No, cholesterol is good. In fact your body actually makes its own cholesterol, which it uses in the manufacture of cell membranes and big, fat, fun hormones.
Q. So are you saying that cholesterol is good then, doctor?
A. No, cholesterol is bad. Cholesterol and blood mix like Paris Hilton and a Mensa meeting. The cholesterol needs some little boats called lipoproteins to ferry cholesterol about the bloodstream. There are "lousy" LDL boats and "healthy" HDL boats, all carrying the cholesterol riders to their various destinations. The lousy LDL ferries are full of nasty, wee, fat passengers that have all gorged themselves at Wong Fung's All-You-Can-Jam-Into-Your-Honorable-Duodenum Szechuan restaurant. These boats have

bumper stickers that read "I Brake For Plaques." The healthy HDL boats, with little bumper stickers that read "I Break Plaques," run around and try and undo the damage done by the LDL ones. It is the ratio of HDL to LDL that makes a huge difference in whether or not your coronary arteries block off. By taking a blood test, we can determine if you have enough good boats to offset the bad guys. If you don't, then according to the fine folks of Framingham, you are at a large risk of waking up dead with a heart attack.

Q. What about genes?

A. Don't wear 'em.

Q. No, I mean, can I inherit high cholesterol?

A. Yes. If, for example, your mother died at age twelve and your dad at age six, and all your family reunions are held in the cardiac ward (and you were christened Angie O'Plasty), then you should check your LDL and HDL levels. One in every five hundred people have genetic predisposition to high cholesterol.

Q. So perhaps I should cut down on my cholesterol ingestion, doc.

A. No, in fact it is the ingestion of saturated fats and trans fats that you should cut down on in order to lower your cholesterol. That means the beef and butter (dairy) fats. Trans fats are what make snacks crunchy, snappy, and hard, but remember, the stiffer your snacks, the stiffer your arteries. Food containing predominantly unsaturated fats, like fish and poultry, can actually lower your bad cholesterol. The other key is to get your HDL boats way up in numbers. This is best done by exercising.

Q. What about drugs?

A. No, thanks.

Q. Er... what I mean is... can drugs lower your LDL or raise your HDL?

A. A class of drugs called statins not only helps lower the LDL (and some even raise the HDL) but has been shown to dramatically reduce fatal heart attacks in patients with heart disease.

Q. Why do you keep referring to me as Q?

A. It's a 007 thing.

HARD SNACKS, HARD ARTERIES

Ever since my childhood, which officially ended three years ago when my wife threw out most of my stuffed animals, my Chia Pet, and all my Tinkertoys, I have wanted to see the Arctic Ocean. My wife's idea of a good vacation, however, involves a place where big brown men in grass skirts play ukeleles made from coconut shells. Knowing her preferences, I explained to her that we were heading to a place where the sun shines all the time (in June). I failed to tell her (true story here) that we were going to the northernmost point of land in the U.S. until we were actually on the way to the airport.

Admittedly, she was none too pleased when she got off the plane in the Eskimo town of Barrow, Alaska. The wind off the Arctic Ocean (at minus ten Fahrenheit) blew her muumuu sideways so straight that I felt compelled to salute; she resembled a taut flag in a windstorm. While she stood with feet frozen to the tundra and Hawaiian Tropic frozen to her nostrils, I felt I'd best seek out the local medical guru and get the local low-down before she thawed out.

I found the medicine man chomping away on a piece of frozen whale blubber, so I spoke to him in my very best Pukiliak: "Korliuk ben Nanook forgaki ulu sitsit." For those of you rusty on rare Eskimo dialects, I had said, basically, "Hello."

"Gak, Dave," he replied—which, interpreted, is, "So, you have come, no doubt, to inquire how we, who exist on a diet of bowhead whale blood, seal oil, and walrus butt, and don't know a vegetable from a cue ball, never get heart attacks or cancer, Dave."

"No," I answered, "I was hoping you could tell me where I could buy some really thick and fuzzy long johns."

But he persisted. "I will tell you that our diet, which is rich in omega-3 fatty acids, is actually healthier than both the Mediterranean and the vegetarian diet. The fat we ingest comes from fish oils or marine mammals. It raises the good type of cholesterol (HDL) in our blood while actually lowering the bad cholesterol (LDL). We eat only unsaturated fats, while you eat the saturated fats. You, I fear, eat the dreaded... trans-fatty acids!"

"I know," I agreed, munching on a peanut butter Twinkie. "Furthermore," I continued, unwrapping a Mr. Big, "the nutritional catchphrase of the year is AVOID TRANS-FATTY ACIDS. Not only do we hydrogenate our fats, but research shows we prefer to eat snacks that are crispy and crunchy. To get our snacks to snap, crackle, and pop, we convert them into trans-fatty acids (TFA). While you use your liquid sunshine oils, we load up our foods with TFAs that stiffen up the product. We eat crackers, french fries, chips, doughnuts, sticks of hard butter, and white bread, all full of it."

"You are indeed full of it," he agreed. "And what really frosts my bearskin shorts is that if we ever start eating your trans-fatty acids and hydrogenated fats, we, too, not only will get more heart disease and cancer but will develop degenerative diseases like arthritis, diabetes and colitis, as well as psoriasis and gallstones. We may become so physically and mentally addled that we will start listening to Howard Stern."

"Yikes," I yiked. "Pass the blubber."

"Wait, though," he cautioned. "If you were to follow an Eskimo diet, you might fare poorly, just as if we Eskimos followed a tropical diet, we, too, might die. You must follow the diet natural to your area."

"Great!" says I. "I live in McWhopperville."

"No, you fliaknook, you must use olive oil rather than butter, you must avoid overprocessed foods, and you must read the label."

I glanced at mine, which read: 100 per cent polyester, Made in Bangladesh.

"No, foolish mukluk. Food labels. They will never actually say 'trans-fatty acid,' but will instead say 'saturated' or 'hydrogenated fats' or even 'vegetable shortening.' Remember that the crispier and stiffer the fats you eat, the crispier and stiffer your arteries become."

Satisfied that I had educated him on the essentials of a civilized diet, I went to retrieve my wife, who I found at a shark cartilage feast surrounded by nervous Eskimo lawyers, discussing the concept of quickie Alaskan divorces. As she bit into her food, I heard an awful cracking, snapping sound. Initially disgusted by the thought of her chomping into some TFAS, I was relieved to discover that it was only the Hawaiian Tropic cracking on her face. Serves her right for tossing out my Tinkertoys.

NUTS TO YOU

On rare occasions, when I find my pantry low on the essential food groups such as Cocoa Puffs, Snickers, and Dr. Pepper, I go grocery shopping. Not one to linger too long in the tofu and wheat germ aisle, I slink over to the bulk food section, salivating fondly over these massive barrels of massive calories. When it comes to the cases of nuts, admittedly, I am a bit of a nutcase. I scoop up a large mixture of nuts, flick aside the ugly Brazil nuts, flick in a few more cashews, and make for my pantry.

But I happen to have two teenage sons/squirrels nesting in my home. By the time I get around to treating myself, I notice that all of the cashews have mysteriously fallen out of the bag. My "Keep your hands off my nuts!" command does nothing but garner snickers, which, as I mentioned, is in fact one of the more important food groups. Returning later, I find the almonds have been selectively extricated and are gone. Finally, the walnuts are freed from the mix, leaving me with nothing but a bag of filberts and salt. This drives me . . . exactly.

Nuts, though unquestionably chock-full of fat, just might be the healthiest snack in your cupboard.

Almonds

A handful of almonds a day will keep the cardiovascular surgeon away. Lowering LDL cholesterol, known as the mother of all evil cholesterol, is essential for routine heart-pump maintenance. In fact, in those who are at risk of heart disease, it's necessary to lower LDL cholesterol aggressively. According to the nutty professors at Harvard who study these things, a daily handful of almonds can lower LDL cholesterol enough to reduce cardiovascular disease by a whopping 20 per cent. In some cases a handful of almonds may be used instead of cholesterol-lowering medication. Almonds are also rich in folate, a vitamin important in keeping hearts, fetuses, bones, and brains healthy.

Cashew!

Gesundheit! These luxurious nuts are nothing to sneeze at. Cashews are rich in selenium, a mineral shown to protect against prostate cancer. (This being the case, my sons should have the healthiest prostates south of Spitsbergen.) Cashews, like most nuts, are best eaten unsalted and raw while the oil is fresh. Like almonds, these nuts are loaded with monounsaturated fats, which is good fat. If "good fat" makes as much sense as "slumber party" or "cat owner," realize that, like good cholesterol, unsaturated fat acts biochemically to reduce the risk of cancers and coronaries.

Walnuts

Rich in omega-3 fatty acids, walnuts are, like fish, beneficial in lowering cholesterol. They are also rich in arginine, an amino acid important in the synthesis of nitric oxide, which helps relax tense blood vessels.

Pistachios

The nuts with the highest density of nutrients and the lowest calories, pistachios can help lower cholesterol and are an excellent source of fiber and Vitamin B6. They are also chock full of lutein, thought to possibly act as a protective antioxidant against the blinding condition known as macular degeneration. But these nuts have been known to cause an unfortunate disease known in the medical field as Pistachio Nail. Wrestling vigorously to get at a pistachio may cause scrapes under the tender thumbnail skin, which, when further irritated with salt, will cause its victim to insert the injured thumb deep into the mouth. Sucking vigorously at the thumb, the victim is often seen simultaneously sifting through the bag for easier pistachios.

Peanuts

Peanuts are not your normal nut. In fact, peanuts are no more a nutcase than Michael Jackson isn't. They are legumes. But as we can salt them, roast them, and sell them in the bulk food containers, let's consider them nuts. The average child will eat 1,500 peanut butter sandwiches by the time they graduate from high school. This is not necessarily bad, as peanuts are high in fiber, niacin, and a powerful antioxidant called resveratrol, the same flavanol that gives red wine its reputation as a protector of hearts. Same benefit, less hangover at recess.

So as I sit here with my bag of filberts and salt, my everlasting-prostate sons are fully sated. While a corn doodle or other empty carb snack leaves the snacker hungry again in thirty minutes, a handful of nuts satisfies hunger pangs for several hours. Nut snackers actually eat less, lose weight, and have less diabetes. Satisfying, fat, tasty, and highly nut—ricious.

DOCTOR SOCKEYE

It came out of nowhere. A hundred-foot gray ocean behemoth lunged out of the fog right toward the boat I was perched on, some twenty-three miles out into the Pacific Ocean.

"Shut off your engine and reel in your rod!" came the orders from the intimidating gray hull of a police ocean cruiser. "You in the bright white shirt, you are fishing in a NO FISH ZONE."

"But. . . but officer, I'm not wearing a bright white shirt."

"Well, then, put a shirt on before we go blind, and let's take a look at your catch."

"Okay, throw me something (snicker). As you can see, I have NO fish in this NO FISH ZONE, so why don't. . ."

"But you were, in fact, fishing. We saw your flasher, and that's all we need to see to give you this 250-dollar ticket."

"Hold on a second, Cap'n High Liner. How was I supposed to know that I drifted into a no-fishing zone? I don't see any signs."

"Check your GPS, guppy. Have a good Friday."

Busted by fish fuzz, carp cops, pickerel police. And I hadn't even caught any salmon. But the day was not to be a total loss. I cruised over into the FISH-YOUR-BRAINS-OUT ZONE and reeled in a lovely large spring salmon, which weighed approximately 36.476 pounds by my guesstimate, though the broken scale at the marina had it pegged at 23. (I know it was broken because many of the other experienced fishermen had also noticed that the numbers on the scales were much different than what the fish actually weighed in their experienced hands.) But my fish was expensive—an extra 250 dollars tagged onto the usual fishing expenses of gas, seasickness pills, seventeen lost lures, one lost lunch, one lost watch, multiple large surgical bandages, skin hook extractor, three bribes, and the requisite purchase of the market's salmon special on the way home.

Was it worth it? Depends on how much value you put on your health.

Most of you within the sound of this book will die of a stroke, a heart attack, cancer, or a naked bungee-jumping accident. Several studies have now confirmed that omega-3 fatty acids lessen the risk factors for stroke and heart attacks, but do very little for cancer or bungee cords. The American Heart Association studies indicate that omega-3s decrease the growth of artery-clogging plaques, thin the blood, and lower the level of those dangerous serum triglycerides, and even appear to lower blood pressure a little. Salmon is drenched in omega-3 fatty acids, something we get little or none of in the typical North American diet.

Q. What about fish being contaminated with ocean residue?

A. Farmed fish do have more contaminants than wild salmon. They are fed fish pellets that may have concentrated PCBs, dioxins, and heavy metal contaminants like mercury and Black Sabbath. Any salmon labeled "Atlantic" is actually farmed. Wild salmon tends to be safer to eat but tougher to catch than farmed. Cooked properly, however, 50 per cent of contaminants can be removed from any fish—farmed, wild, or pet.

Q. What about fish oil supplements?

A. Fish oil is considered safe, as any contaminants are usually removed during processing. However, it lacks some of the other beneficial ingredients contained in real fish, including several nutrients and many of my most expensive lures.

Q. So what do you recommend?

A. Two servings of fish per week is the current recommendation, but if you are at high risk for cardiovascular disease, you might consider supplements as well, after consulting with your doctor. Fish oils, for example, can mess up Coumadin, a common heart drug used to thin the blood. Osteoporosis clinics will often take patients off fish oil high in vitamin A, a compound that adversely affects bone density.

And most importantly, I recommend you never expose your flasher to the fish fuzz on Friday.

GO AND SIN-DROME NO MORE

Most of you began reading this book feeling healthy and happy. My job today is to make you feel otherwise. Twenty-five per cent of you will close this chapter sicker than before you started it, diagnosed with a new medical condition you were blissfully unaware you had. So it might be prudent of you to stop reading now and fast-forward to some of the more pleasant aspects of this book, like the back cover. Then make a wee bonfire of the book, feel terribly guilty, and go and purchase another. Repeat until the folks at Pulitzer take notice.

In 1900 the average life expectancy in North America was

forty-seven. Thanks primarily to the likes of vaccination, anti-biotics, and Suzanne Somers, our life expectancy has now increased to seventy-four (unless you happen to be a pedestrian in the vicinity of my newly licensed sons). But now, for the first time ever, we're seeing a projected decrease in life expectancy for those born today compared with those born a generation ago. The reason: many of us unknowingly have metabolic syndrome.

Metabolic sin-drome, as in the sin of gluttony, increases morbidity and mortality.

Even Moses commanded, to the best of my recollection, *Thou shalt not increase thy girth innumerable cubits by gorging thyself at the manna buffet.*

Metabolic syndrome is a precursor to diabetes, which in turn is a precursor to heart attacks and strokes, which are precursors to death, which is a precursor to being reincarnated possibly as an armadillo, and WHO THE HECK WANTS TO BE THAT?

There are five vital facts about your health that you should be able to recite cold: your fasting blood sugar, your HDL, your triglycerides, your blood pressure, and your belt size. Should I approach you on the beach and say, "Quick, tell me your HDL," you should be able to respond immediately with something other than "Officer!"

If you have any *three* of the following five problems, then you have metabolic sin-drome, a nasty diagnosis that does not bode well for the quality or the quantity of your future.

1. Fasting blood sugar above 6.1 mmol/L (millimoles per liter). While 6.1 is not quite sweet enough to be considered diabetic, it is knocking on the door.
2. Triglycerides greater than 1.7 mmol/L. These are your serum fat levels, also known as your Krispy Kreme count.
3. HDL cholesterol less than 1 mmol/L in men and 1.3 mmol/L in women. HDL is the good (happy) cholesterol that can be increased through regular exercise.

4. Hypertension, specifically a blood pressure consistently greater than 130 over 85.

5. Belt size greater than forty inches in men and thirty-five inches in women. Increasing the length of your belt means decreasing the length of your life. Eighty-five per cent of pre-diabetics are overweight or obese, the so-called "diabesity" iceberg so prevalent in North America.

Depending on your gender, you should be able to quote these vital statistics as readily as your wedding date or Steve Nash's field goal percentage on Thursdays. Determining the first four items on the above list requires a visit to a good doctor; the last, a visit to an honest tailor.

Simply having three of five puts you at four times the risk of having a heart attack or stroke. You may feel perfectly fine, with perhaps the only symptom being a touch of laziness, but under the surface is an iceberg about to bring down the HMS *You*.

So please, don't get diabetes, and try to avoid its precursor, metabolic syndrome. It is primarily your decision whether or not you are going to be diabetic. If you do have metabolic syndrome, then you need treatment, in the form of medication and lifestyle change. Learning to "make the healthy choice the easy choice" is the key to lifestyle change. For example, having healthy food like vegetables, fruits, and Snickers in the house rather than pizza, chips, and kale makes it easy to make the right choice when the midnight snacker invades your pang center. Current gas prices may be a blessing in disguise if it makes us get out of our Explorers and Pathfinders and start exploring and finding paths for our Super Flyer two-wheeler. Making 150 minutes of exercise a week needs to be a priority.

Now go and sin-drome no more.

MOUNT ATHEROMA

While living on the remote and primitive island of Tanna in Vanuatu in 1995, my four fearless/feisty/foolish kids and I ventured up the side of a large, nasty volcano named Mount Yasur. This volcano is so dangerous that, were it located in any place in the world other than Tanna, we'd not be allowed within two time zones of it. But there, nobody cares how stupid you are, and being second to no one in that category, I edged up the peak to peek over the edge and into the Earth's fiery furnace.

While we stood/cowered/bargained with the Lord there, the earth beneath our feet suddenly gave a mighty groan. Yasur first rumbled, then belched, and then, to the great alarm of our souls/minds/bladders, it suddenly exploded with a terrifying bellow!

We fell to the ground, certain that we were about to be shot heavenward/dumped into the river Styx. Massive lava boulders the size of Cadillacs/Rhode Island/John Daly flew straight up over our heads. They seemed to hover in mid-air for a moment and then, throttled by gravity, came crashing back, falling either into the boiling cauldron or onto the ground where we lay quivering like frightened felines.

No sooner did we retrieve our mercury/amalgam/dentures than it exploded again! We flew/scurried/cartwheeled down the mountainside as fast as forty pounds of goosebumps clinging to our carcasses would allow. While stumbling down the slope, dodging the meteor shower, we vowed to never return. Mount Yasur claimed three lives during the time I lived at its base and at its mercy.

While I had the sobering opportunity to live in the South Pacific's infamous "ring of fire," many of you may have the sobering realization that a ring of fire lives in *you*. A string of volcanoes, many ready to erupt, rumble within our arterial system, with a particularly dense collection lining our coronary and cerebral arteries. Known as atheroma, these volcanoes are the number one cause of death in the civilized world.

"Atheroma" comes from the Greek for "porridge." I can still hear my sweet, wee Scottish gran, "Eat yer bloody atheroma 'ere yer kilt'll fall down about yer lily-white ankles, exposin' yer lily-white... umm... knickers," which of course is something no self-respecting son of Scotland could bear. The core of the atheroma is a porridge-like, soft, lipid-rich material built up by too much LDL cholesterol. The volcano is covered by a fibrous cap that keeps it from erupting. This sclerotic (hard) fibrous cap is what causes "hardening of the arteries," a condition also known as atherosclerosis.

This cap, however, is eroded by infections (like gingivitis), high blood pressure, and even smoking, which can shear the cap right off. The rupture of Mount Atheroma into the bloodstream is plugged by platelets and sticky buns, which clot over the volcano, seemingly a good thing. But no! In a classic case of the fix being worse than the problem, it is this clot that kills. The rupture/clot is so large that it shuts off all blood flow in the artery, giving its owner a heart attack or stroke.

Soon Mr. LDL Bloggins is getting his photo in the local paper, followed by several kind phrases he never heard in life that include the words "beloved"/"suddenly"/"probate." So keep yer cap on, and keep yer porridge in yer tummy, not yer bloodstream.

FLOSS FANGS FREQUENTLY

It was a dark and stormy night that ushered me into a dark and stormy hut in the far reaches of a dark jungle island in the stormy South Pacific. There he sat, his dark Melanesian eyes riveted on my stormy face, eyes that likely had seldom, if ever, set sight upon an extremely white man. Pointing to his mouth, he mumbled, in obvious discomfort, "*Mrgghshslprr*," which translated means "I've got a tooth that's driving me to extraction."

Living on a jungle isle, far from civilization and Regis Philbin, I had become, as the only doctor to 30,000 people, a jack of all medical specialties. So why not dentist? Nothing dentured, nothing gained, and besides, how tough could it be? Stuff one inflated balloon in patient's mouth, stretch upper lip over eyebrows and lower lip to navel, hum elevator music, discuss athletic prowess of my children, and draw up a bill equivalent to the GNP of Burkina Faso. Grabbing the anesthetic needle, I tried to remember how my dentist had managed to freeze my tooth, along with my lip, nostrils, and dandruff. I muttered the bush surgeon's motto, "I'm not really sure how to do this, but I'm the best around." And I did freeze his tooth!—and his nostrils and his vocal cords, and for that matter, the entire left side of his body.

"*Blagggrrkaak*," he moaned, which translated means, "Did I just have a stroke?" I proceeded to extricate this rotten but nonetheless tough little tooth. I wiggled and twisted, cursed and prayed, pushed, pulled, pried, prodded, begged, and cursed some more. A puddle of sweat appeared on the floor, some of it mine. Finally, much to the relief of the two of us, I yanked out the prize, a sugarcane-rotted package of dentin and enamel.

Little did I realize, according to a study out of Harvard University, that I was dramatically increasing this fellow's risk of having a stroke, not by my method of applying anesthesia but rather by reducing his quota of teeth. This intriguing study indicated that men with fewer than twenty-five teeth, i.e., the Boston Bruins (cumulative), had a whopping 57 per cent higher risk of stroke than those with more than twenty-five teeth. I will pause now and allow you time to run to the mirror to count your teeth.

Hello again.

Most of us are headed for a stroke, heart attack, or cancer. According to the obituary pages and my practice, most of us will use one of these three vehicles to exit this planet, Shirley MacLaine and Raëlians excepted. Some of course will show up in these pages as a result of slipping on a banana peel while participating in the Silverback Gorilla Prostate Study, but for most of us, our families will be asking for donations to societies with the word "vascular" in their name.

For years, my dentist has reminded me that poor dental hygiene can lead to serious and sudden cardiovascular disease. For years, my dentist has reminded me to sit still, put down Pooh Bear, and quit sniveling.

Periodontal disease appears to create a nasty inflammation in the arteries. This inflammation increases the accumulation of arterial plaque. This plaque can break off and head to the heart, where it precipitates a heart attack, or to the brain, where it causes a stroke. Dr. Don Smith, director of the Colorado Neurological Institute, warns, "Good dental hygiene may achieve the level of importance in stroke prevention that we now accord to control blood pressure, cessation of smoking, exercise, and healthy diet." Though the precise mechanism has yet to be determined, a high correlation exists between those with gingivitis or the more severe periodontitis and stroke and heart attacks.

So for fewer fatalities, floss your fangs frequently.

Plaque building up in your teeth may well reflect plaque building up in your arteries. From one plaque to another. Mi plaqua su plaqua. Quid pro quo, Clarissa. E pluribus unum.

If all of this talk of heart attacks and dentists and *mrgghshslprr* and Regis seems a little disjointed and rambling, please be patient. I'm a little long in the tooth.

STROKE OF LUCK

Walter, a wiry and robust fifty-two-year-old who bops through life as if his diet consists purely of Jolt, dill pickles, and lemon juice, bounced out to the farmhouse, intent on whitewashing the cellar of the old place. Suddenly his head began to throb. He'd been plagued with headaches most of his life, but nothing like this. Alarmed, he headed back home and tried to explain what was happening, but words failed him like George W.

Have you guessed what Walter's problem was? Fortunately, his family recognized that healthy Walter was having a stroke, and they rushed him to the hospital. His type of stroke required emergency surgery if he was to stand a chance of surviving, an outcome his family was warned likely would not happen. But he did survive.

When he awoke, however, Walter had no memory of the past twenty years, including the fact that his son Wayne was the greatest hockey player in the world. Walter Gretzky now devotes no small part of his borrowed time traveling to assorted heart and stroke conventions, warning us all to be aware of the symptoms of stroke.

Will you be one of the 170,000 North Americans *under* age sixty-five or one of the 330,000 sixty-five and older who will have a stroke this year? Risk factors include all the usual suspects we've come to hate: obesity, smoking, high cholesterol, high blood pressure, diabetes, dancing the Macarena, etc.

Know the five signs of a stroke! Pin these to your fridge, furniture, or forehead.

1. Speech difficulties, finding a word or articulatering it
2. Disturbance of vision, as in sudden loss or doubling of
3. Headache—sudden, severe, and unusual
4. Weakness or numbness/tingling, usually only on one side of your body
5. Dizziness leading to a sudden fall or unsteadiness

Memorize these five symptoms. The mnemonic SDHWD helps, as in Send Dave Hepburn Wads of Dough. Repeat this mantra until it becomes a part of your very being.

Fifteen per cent of all strokes are a result of a brain artery bursting, most often as a result of high blood pressure. Eighty-five per cent of strokes are caused by the clogging of a brain artery, either through Big Mac plaque buildup or from wee clots being shot off from an irregularly beating heart. If you can get a stroke victim to a proper stroke facility quickly and the clot is busted within three hours, about a third of these patients will recover with no disability. But the longer brain tissue is deprived of blood, the more apt a patient is to end up writing books like these ones. TIME IS BRAIN.

For years, not much could be done for stroke victims, but now many new and exciting treatment options exist. The greatest success is with the new clot busters including tPA and even Ancrod, the venom of the Malaysian pit viper. The snake simply latches on to your arm and injects its clot-busting venom. (Just kidding, it actually latches on to your neck.)

A TIA (transient ischemic attack) is a warning that you are about to have a stroke in the next few days or weeks. Generally lasting less than one hour, TIAS may consist of any of the above five symptoms, which by now you have memorized using the mnemonic I taught you (please repeat this SDHWD each and every time you head to the... umm... bank). Get seen immediately, even if these symptoms clear up, as a TIA precedes a stroke.

Does your city have a dedicated Stroke Unit attached to the hospital? If not, YOU NEED ONE. Why? Because when it comes time for you to have your stroke, you will want it treated within the allotted time and by a dedicated "brain attack team" that's ready and eager to kick some clot. Remember that dying at age ninety-five is okay, but living at age fifty-five after having been felled by a disabling stroke is rough.

As for Walter Gretzky, though he has recovered, he has been left with some serious memory deficits. Try as he might, he just can't seem to recall that Wayne and I were separated at birth.

PRESSURE WATCHER

After a patient has waited the customary twenty-seven minutes in an exam room, preceded by the customary fifty-two minutes in the waiting room (hence the term "patient"), I am curious to see how they've bided their time, especially when kids are involved. In a room replete with scientific discovery, kids are often found reflexing with the reflex hammer, jamming tongue depressors into various orifices their teddy bear didn't realize he even had, or giving injections to a wailing sister. Mom, meanwhile, is deeply engrossed in the office's latest *Time* magazine (i.e., the annexation of Alaska). But the kids' single-greatest source of entertainment is the blood pressure cuff, commonly known, of course, as the sphyngomanometer. They just love to get that thing wrapped around their mother's forearm or their brother's neck, pumping the wee bulb as vigorously as their meaty little paws can pump.

Why is it that every MD's office has a blood pressure cuff? A doctor may lack rubber gloves, matching socks, or a medical degree, but he never lacks for a BP cuff. Is blood pressure all that important to doctors? Indeed, it is.

Also known as the silent killer, high blood pressure is so insidious that you may go to bed feeling perfectly perky but wake to discover you are dead. Are you one of the estimated 20 million North Americans who are hypertensive but unaware of it? Will you find out you were hypertensive after you've suffered your first stroke? Perhaps it will be a heart attack, heart failure, or kidney failure that will alert you to the fact that you should've checked your BP every year. As high blood pressure percolates over the years it doesn't turn your ears red, bulge out your eyes, or cause any pain. Then suddenly, it hurts a lot.

The commonest cause of hypertension is called "essential hypertension," meaning essentially we don't know what causes it. We are, however, aware of some predisposing risk factors, including:

· Obesity and lack of exercise. Exercising fifty minutes four times a week is the equivalent of taking one whole blood pressure-lowering pill!

· High salt intake, 80 per cent of which comes from salty foods like pickles, chips, and saltlicks.

· Stress. One study showed that young adults who were stressed were 7.5 times more likely to develop hypertension ten years later!

- Smoking. No doubt all the smokers who read health books are shocked to realize this.
- Alcohol. Keep to a maximum of one day per glass, bub.
- Age. Systolic blood pressure tends to rise with age, but diastolic pressure tends to drop.

The systolic pressure (the first number) is the pressure in your system when the pump (your heart) is fully contracted. The higher the systolic, the higher the risk of stroke. We like to see this number below 140, REGARDLESS OF AGE! Some doctors do not treat the systolic pressure adequately in the elderly because they feel that the diastolic number is fine or even low. Whoops.

The diastolic (second number) is the pressure in your system when the heart relaxes between beats. If it is too high, then the risk of heart disease, kidney failure, and stroke increases. Reducing diastolic pressure by as little as five points can mean a 40 per cent reduction in stroke risk and a 50 per cent reduction in heart failure.

One problem in determining blood pressure is that the doctor's office may not be the most appropriate place to take a reading. Whitecoat hypertension is a very common entity that can cause a BP to read thirty points higher in a doctor's office than it would at home. The patient finds himself in the office of the purveyor of pain, deliverer of doom, and bearer of bad breath. The preceding patient has just left the office, screaming in pain and carrying an ear. The walls seem to yell, "Quick, get out of here!" This is hardly conducive to a normal pressure. I am, therefore, a proponent of home monitors. It's much more effective, both fiscally and medically, to put our effort into detecting and treating the blood pressure problem than trying to treat the consequences of neglect.

Hypertension is the third leading cause of death worldwide, behind malnutrition and tobacco. So please, go and get your pressure taken somewhere. If you refuse, I'm sending the kids by to check you over.

STAY AHEAD OF THE GAME

On a recent hockey junket to southern Alberta, I found myself (appropriately for a hockey tournament) in the community of Head-Smashed-In Buffalo Jump. That night, I slept fitfully at the Head-Smashed-In Inn, no doubt apprehensive about having to play a team called Head-Smashed-In Trauma Kings. Team Motto: "If you can't beat 'em, just beat 'em." In fact, I had nothing to fear, as I was more at risk of head injury driving to the rink than I was actually playing the game. Of all head injuries, only 10 per cent are a result of recreational activity (attending N.Y. Ranger home games excluded). Falls account for 21 per cent, violence (attending N.Y. Rangers home games included) for 12 per cent, and a whopping 50 per cent from motor vehicle accidents.

The brain sloshes happily about inside the human skull, bathed in cerebrospinal fluid (CSF). It spends most of its day snapping off synaptic signals, controlling bodily functions, and playing condescending mind games with the kidneys. "Hey kiddies, hurry up and piddle so we can go to the Stones concert tonight and... oh, wait... ha... kidney stones!"

When the head receives a sudden jolt, the skull comes to an abrupt stop. The brain, which should have been watching the road rather than analyzing its emotional response to the blond hitchhiker, actually smacks into the inside wall of the skull. This causes a stunning (concussion), bruising (contusion), bleeding (bleeding), or a sudden decrease of intellect (urge to play hockey). "Hey brainiac," tease the kidneys, "keep your eye on the road, or urine trouble."

Two things concern us when you crack your cranium.

1. Concussion

Having your brain smacked and swollen may lead to confusion, loss of consciousness, and memory loss, rendering you prime material as a senator. The duration of unconsciousness or of the memory bank being closed for service is an indication of how bad the concussion is. A subsequent concussion (even minor), if incurred before the first one heals properly, can lead to dire consequences. After "having your bell rung," do not risk a re-injury to the head unless cleared by a doctor. Unless raised downwind of Three Mile Island, you have only one head, and damage caused by concussion can be permanent.

2. *Bleeding*

A leaking blood vessel inside the skull is an emergency. When the brain sloshes around the skull after a collision it may shear a vein, allowing a slow leak, or it may shear an artery, leading to a more drastic bleed. The skull is rigid but the brain is soft. As pressure increases inside the skull, the brain gets compressed even to the point of being forced down your neck! This is usually a major bummer.

A visit to the doctor will prompt ol' Sawbones to grab an instrument called an eye looker-inner. He will place this to his eye and then thrust his face so close to yours, you'll be able to trade eyelash lice. This prompts an intense giggle reflex in the patient, who will snort and struggle not to breathe. Besides checking to make sure the pupils are equal, the doctor is actually shining the light into the back of the eye. He is not examining the eye itself. Rather, this is the only place in the entire human body where he can directly examine blood vessels, nerves, and the oompa loompas running around inside your skull. What he sees will tell him if any significant pressure is being built up inside the cranium.

Assuming all appears okay, he will then send you home with a list of symptoms to watch for, including:

1. Protracted vomiting.
2. Unremitting headache that doesn't clear with Tylenol.
3. Vision blurring as one pupil becomes larger than the other.
4. Acting bizarrely. This is the most important symptom of brain damage, and includes such irrational behavior as dating Hugh Hefner (what a waste of perfectly good blonds) or planning your next hockey trip to...Wounded Knee Buffalo Jump.

A SHAKY START TO THE OLYMPICS

Having dashed headlong down the stadium ramp, we herded ourselves around the track at Atlanta's Centennial Olympic Stadium, waving to dignitaries, assorted dictators, and the coup plotters sitting beside them. As team doctor, interpreter, and token white guy, I was part of the Olympic team for the powerhouse nation Vanuatu (no medals, like, *ever*) in the 1996 Olympics. After coming to a disorganized halt in the infield, we gazed up into the hot Atlanta night toward the yet unlit Olympic torch. Weeks of speculation about who would be the chosen one to light the Olympic flame was about to be extinguished.

Suddenly, a large figure appeared on the steps. I recognized him immediately as Al the security guard, who earlier had confiscated my camera, firecrackers, and Pepsi (this was the Coke Olympics). I then glanced over to where everyone else was staring slack-jawed, to witness a tremulous Muhammad Ali perched precariously high above the stadium. Both his flame and his frame were waving madly in the sky.

The next day, as I sat in the Olympic cafeteria between the Chinese and Mexican sections, Muhammad Ali wheeled into the hall accompanied by his wife, Lonnie. The entire cafeteria stood and applauded. Lonnie told me later that Ali's shaky start to the Olympics was due in part to his distaste for taking his medication.

Muhammad Ali has Parkinson's Disease (PD).

Caused by the death of cells in a part of the brain called the substantia nigra, PD unfortunately afflicts more than a million of our fellow North Americans. PD is not yet diagnosed by a blood test, but rather by detecting two of the following three symptoms:

- A tremor that only occurs when the arm or hand is at rest, but disappears with intentional movement. Ali, for example, displayed no shaking as he reached over with the torch to light the cauldron. But, had he held the flickering inferno in his hand while resting for any length of time, Hotlanta might've be Shermanized once more. Be advised that not all tremors are PD. Tremors can be a symptom of many conditions, including thyroid disease, anxiety, or drinking Jolt on a jackhammer job.

· Rigidity of limbs and muscles. Not always obvious, many cases of PD rigidity have been misdiagnosed as tennis elbow or a stiff arm, particularly in younger patients.

· A slowing of voluntary movement, including walking. Tim Conway's old-man shuffle is the classic gait of PD.

These symptoms often conspire to create other classic signs of PD, including the deterioration of writing skills (approaches MD quality in severe cases), monotonous speech (approaches Al Gore in severe cases), and a decrease in facial expressions with infrequent blinking (approaches my old babysitter, Mrs. Robocop).

While Parkinson's is generally considered an old person's disease, an alarming 30 per cent of those with PD now present before the age of fifty! The most publicized of this group is the youthful Michael J. Fox, who has remained seventeen years old for the past twenty years.

What causes Parkinson's? Perhaps pesticides, metals, viruses, lack of Vitamin D, genes, or putting your skull through the Thrilla in Manila are causes, but nothing has yet been proven.

It is known that the cells that die in PD are those that produce dopamine, a vital neurotransmitter. While "L-dopa" may sound like Zorro's drugged-out sidekick, it is, in fact, the mainstay drug for treating the symptoms of Parkinson's. Surgery can also now be performed in select patients to alleviate PD's tremor aspect. A stimulating probe is inserted into a part of the brain that controls tremors, and a battery is then installed under the skin of the chest in order to keep the probe working. Michael J. Fox underwent such a procedure. Finally, clinical trials are also underway to define the role of stem cells and nerve cell transplants into the brain.

We'd all love to see the DeLorean up and running again.

YOU-GOTTA-QUIT-YOU-GOTTA-QUIT-YOU-GOTTA-QUIT

We have a new dog. This yearling lab cross is not exactly the crispiest Milk-Bone in the box. For starters, this pup insists on sticking his beak under the couch, from which our ill-tempered cat, Shere Khan, rules the house. Repeatedly, the cat employs the pup's snout as a scratching post. Repeatedly, this ditzy dog insists on peering under the couch to see if by some miracle the cat has had a change of heart.

But by far the best indication that this dog comes from a long line of incest is his incessant tail chasing. A simple tweak of the tail sends this dog into a whirling dervish spin for several minutes. As the RPMs pick up, our pirouetting puppy spins himself like a figure skater on Jolt.

"I'm-gonna-get-it-I'm-gonna-get-it-I'm-gonna-get-it-I'm-gonna-get-it-Whoa-I'm-dizzy-I'm-gonna-get-it-I'm-gonna-get-it-I'm-gonna-get-it." After landing with an awkward splat on the floor, he up and heads right over to check under the couch—where, no doubt, the cat has been laughing up a hairball. "Hey, puss, bet you haven't seen spinning action like that bef. . ."

"Pffffffttt!"

Similar tail chasing occurs in medicine.

"You-gotta-quit-smoking-you-gotta-quit-smoking-you-gotta-quit-smoking-Paul-is-dead-you-gotta-quit-smoking-you-gotta-quit-smoking-you-gotta-quit-smoking." Cigarette smokers cause our medical system to chase our "butts" until we fall with a splat. Some cardiovascular surgeons, for example, actually refuse to operate on a patient's smoking-related circulatory problems unless the patient stops the ruinous behavior that got him or her there.

FACT: It has been calculated that *each* cigarette smoked whittles eleven minutes off a smoker's life! Think of the waste. Even a single puff could cost you the time you would have spent watching *George W's Insightful Thoughts* video.

Okay, if you're in your seventies (i.e., Britney Spears is a type of asparagus from the north of France), then you could *almost* be excused for having a smoking problem. Not only was smoking acceptable way back when, but doctors even recommended the occasional puff to help treat stress. We now know, however, that smoking actually *causes* stress. Stress levels rise and stay high upon hearing, "Bloggins, you have cancer of the (select one or more of: lung, esophagus, bladder, stomach, throat, mouth, and likely many more of your favorite organs)."

But what really gets doctors fuming is trying to figure out why those of you who have grown up aware of the destructive effects of smoking do it anyway. Doctors don't agree on much, but we've all seen the incredibly harmful effects of smoking. We wonder what goes through smokers' minds when they open up a package decorated with skull and crossbones and assorted dire warnings. What part of the word "death" is so difficult to figure out? Would you buy cat food for your cat if the package label included "WARNING: This cat food may kill your cat"?

So time to butt out. How? Popular quitting methods include:

1. The patch. Once the most popular method, the nicotine patch slowly reduces the body's dependence on the most addictive of the three thousand chemicals inhaled when smoking. Works best when placed directly over the mouth.

2. Hypnotism. It may occasionally be helpful, but side effects include stripping naked and crowing like a rooster each time someone claps their hands and yells, "Muskrat!"

3. Pills. These have the highest success rate by far. The most exciting of these medications actually mimics nicotine's pleasurable effects while blocking the smoked nicotine from doing anything. I have heard two-pack-a-day-for-forty-year smokers state that this medication makes smoking a cigarette seem like smoking air. They quit.

But others must be terribly worried about their health. "So, what are the side effects of this pill, doctor?" Bloggins inquires, coughing and hacking as though the alien is about to explode out of his chest. This has always struck me as one of the more absurd questions I hear.

"What do you care, Bloggins? You smoke!"

"Well, I just like to be careful about my health, you know."

"Okay, one out of every 700,000 people will get a zit on their left kneecap."

"Left, eh? Well, I'm not so sure I want to risk. . ." (cough, sputter, hacks up emphysematous lung)

"To be honest, it doesn't matter if it causes your left ear to fall off. Would you like to review the side effects of smoking, Bloggins?"

"Well, I really can't afford the fifty dollars per month."

"Of course not. You're paying 150 dollars per month to have your health go up in smoke. The 1800 dollars you burn this year could be used to buy a week's worth of gas or a couple of Knicks tix."

"Well, sounds good, doctor, but I'm just-not-ready-just-not-ready-just-not-ready-just-not-ready-hey-it's-the-Grim-Reaper-just-not-ready-just—"

• • •

I'D LIKE
(*to* BUY *a*)
BOWEL

• • •

DR. GERD

I hated my nickname as a kid. "Heartburn" was the cruel replacement for Hepburn. "Hey, Heartburn, wanna belch the alphabet?" I was sure that this nickname cost me tons of chicks. I seriously considered changing to my mother's maiden name of Hemmings until I realized that hemmorrhoid would not be a vast improvement on heartburn. And so I was stuck with this witty moniker of teenagerdom. I have hated the word heartburn ever since.

Even to this day, when questioning a patient, I refuse to ask if they suffer heartburn. Instead, I inquire, "Have you noticed any gastroesophageal reflux disease (GERD)?"

"What?"

"You know, acid reflux."

"You mean heartburn, doc?" <wince>

And yet, heartburn <cringe> has been the story of one of my two greatest triumphs as an intern, the other involving a Volkswagen, a nurse nicknamed Sarge, and a flagpole. While still under the watchful eye of an experienced MD preceptor, while working in his office, I met one of his patients, fifty-five-year-old Vern Davis (nicknamed VD).

"My problem, doctor, is that I have a chronic cough, and I'm constantly clearing my throat," he said. Over the years, VD had undergone assorted X-rays, and had been put on various cough medicines and inhalers for his lungs. He'd had allergy tests and sinus treatment, all to no avail. I guess he thought I was his one "last gasp."

It was one of those rare moments in my career when the penny dropped, the kernels popped, the lightbulb lit, the trout finally bit, the hula hooped, and the beetle pooped. I surmised that his lungs and throat were not the source of his cough and irritated throat. Perhaps he had heartb... er... acid reflux. I suggested to the preceptor that we might treat him for GERD. A month later, VD returned, excited to be free of his plague for the first time in years. Now, in my own practice, VD visits me regularly, so to speak.

Although 40 per cent of us suffer from occasional heartbu... GERD, for 7 per cent of North Americans, acid reflux is a daily discomfort. Having, in fact, nothing to do with the heart, burning pain in the chest occurs when the highly acidic stomach contents slide up out of the stomach and into the esophagus or gullet. While the very thick and protective stomach lining can usually deal with this powerful hydrochloric acid, the sensitive esophagus cannot. In addition to digesting food, the acid starts to digest the esophagus. Over time, this problem can lead to severe erosion and on occasion, a very nasty cancer of the esophagus.

The stomach is separated from the esophagus and the chest cavity by means of a bulge of muscle known as the LES or lower esophageal sphincter (nicknamed Lester). When this sphincter doesn't stay taut and protect the esophagus, acid sneaks up from the stomach into the chest and we have hea... GERD. This LES is compromised by diet and posture. Cigarettes, alcohol, coffee (decaf included), peppermint, tomatoes, spices, carbonated drinks, and chocolate all contribute to the acid reflux problem. Frequent bending, tight clothes, pregnancy, obesity, and eating large meals also aggravate it.

"Doc, the wife tells me I got a high-anus hernia," Bloggins explained while pointing to his chest.

"Bloggins, if it hurts in your chest, I'd say it was an extremely high-anus hernia. Perhaps you mean hiatus hernia."

Malapropisms aside, hiatus hernia describes how the top part of the stomach slides or herniates itself up above the diaphragm muscle and into the chest cavity. When this occurs, the Lester weakens and stomach acid can easily create havoc in the esophagus.

Treating GERD includes:

1. Avoiding the diet listed above. Replace with copious amounts of gummy bears.
2. Never eating within three hours of retiring to bed, as GERD develops easily at night.
3. Raising the head of the bed six inches by placing some blocks or books or the cat under the legs at the head of the bed. Your head should be six inches higher than your tail. This remarkably simple maneuver can lead to pain-free sleep.
4. Testing for and treating *H. pylori*, a bacterium that many GERD patients harbor in their stomachs.
5. Taking one of the very effective medications now available that can reduce the acid production or even tighten the LES.
6. Undergoing surgery as a last resort. Like many surgeries these days, it can now be performed via a small keyhole incision. The sphincter is up and running again, so to speak.

If all else fails, see me, Dr. Gerd.

HELICO DANGER

I fly helicopters, or at least I *flew* helicopters, er... I mean I flew one once. Okay, I sat in the cockpit, but I felt like I was flying it. Fine, then, I had a couple of extra quarters and was stranded outside a grocery store. While a medical officer in the Canadian navy ("Yes, Virginia...") during Desert Storm/Gulf War One/ Persian Excursion, I was transported from ship to ship via the infamous Sea King helicopters, better described as 100,000 parts hopefully moving somewhat in tandem.

When a medical situation required that the doctor be transferred from one ship to another, I would be carefully lowered to the quarterdeck on a winch from the helicopter. I'd dash off to sick bay, stitch up the crew, or sober up the captain, and then be retrieved by the helo. Being winched down from a Sea King onto a pitching deck in the middle of the night was tricky at the best of times. But one harrowing day, while being lowered, the winch stopped some twenty-five feet above the deck, too far for me to unharness and jump. All at once the helicopter moved sideways, and within a few moments I was no longer over the deck but was dangling over the salty Persian Gulf, an inhospitable body of water full of sea snakes, box jellyfish, and the usual explosive mines. Suddenly, the winch rapidly let go, making me one of the few men to literally serve my country *in* the Persian Gulf.

As I was systematically submerged into the water and then raised up again gasping for air, I glanced up at the pilots, who were laughing like drunken sailors... (sorry, that's now politically incorrect)... like drunken pilots. Hernias popped out their groins and rum spurted from their nostrils. Then they dropped me again and again until either their fuel or their rum ran out, a game they called "dunking the doctor."

To this day, when a patient comes into the office with "I wanna get tested for that helicopter bug in my stomach," I get a nostalgic taste of Saddam's seawater in my throat.

Helicobacter pylori has become one of the most infamous bacteria of modern times. Since its discovery, it has not only completely changed the way doctors treat stomach ulcers, but it has made us sit up and look at other bacteria and viruses as the possible cause of many diseases that were previously considered mysteries. From arthritis to MS and from Crohn's disease to ADHD and even heart attacks and cancer, more research is focusing on investigating infectious etiology.

H. pylori is a spiral-shaped bacterium that gets dunked deep into our unpleasant stomach fluids. Rather than coming up out of this inhospitable environment gasping for air, it chooses to burrow into the lining of the stomach wall. There it may sit and do nothing, or it may create an inflammatory mess that leads to an irritated gastritis, ulcers, or even gastric cancer. Twenty per cent of the population under age forty harbors hundreds of happy herds of *Helicobacter* in their stomachs. Most do not develop ulcers or stomach cancer, but some do.

H. pylori is likely acquired in childhood when we tend to eat anything and everything other than what is actually put on our plate. Our stomachs were too full of kitty litter, moldy couch peanuts, and whatever was in the dog's dish to bother with Gerber's pureed peach porridge or that contemptible creamed carrot.

Usually *Helicobacter* causes no symptoms, in which case it is not considered a real problem. But the lining of the stomach may become irritated and inflamed to the point it causes burning, belching, bloating, nausea, gas, abdominal distention, and halitosis. While you may have always thought that these symptoms were yet another disgusting family trait, they may, in fact, be caused by a bug. *H. pylori* can be eradicated with appropriate treatment in one week.

Many years ago, as an intern, I assisted in a surgery that was meant to remove a mystery mass from the abdomen of a young man in his thirties. After opening up the abdomen, the surgeon surveyed the mess the mass had made. So much cancer had spread about the abdomen that he said sadly, "I can do nothing. Let's just close him up." I still remember that chilling introduction to gastric cancer.

Gastric carcinoma is the second most frequent cancer worldwide and the number-one cancer killer in many countries, particularly in Asia. Each year 25,000 North Americans are diagnosed with gastric carcinoma, most presenting in the late stages and therefore with poor prognosis.

H. pylori is actually now listed as a human carcinogen, and it may be just about as dangerous as... drunken pilots.

GAS LEAK

My daughter, appreciating my elite level of sophistication, bought me the bestest gift I've ever received. It is only a small black box about the size of, say, a square black kumquat, but it has enriched my life immensely. Known as the GAS TANK, this little device emits realistically rude reverberations simulating sounds that, shall we say, might follow a feast at Bob's Boston Beanery. More than a mere electronic whoopee cushion, this marvel of modern technology comes equipped with a variety of authentic-sounding eruptions, a driver's-side airbag, and, most importantly for me, a remote control.

I find I use this device more often than I do a stethoscope. That's just the innovative type of doctor I am. To the chagrin of Louisa, my receptionist, I use it most at work. On occasion, temptation overtakes me, and I surreptitiously plant this device at her desk among all her death certificates, biopsy specimens, and Twinkies. Then, when the waiting room is packed full of patient patients patiently waiting their turn to be a patient, my evil inner child, with diabolical intent, zaps the zapper from afar and witnesses the sounds and sights that only loud, unexpected flatulence can bring.

I've recently halted this practice, however, since Louisa has developed a nasty tick of her left eyelid, and our clinic's vault of Valium has vanished. But stopping this frivolity cold turkey was causing horrible withdrawal symptoms for me.

So, while attending a course on medical dignity or ethics, or some other trivial nonsense ordered by the judge, with twenty other distinguished colleagues, I caved in. I slipped the wee kumquat into a coat pocket that had been resting innocently on

the back of a chair. I slunk over to the other side of the room
and feigned interest in the lecture. At a relatively quiet moment
in the lecture... ZAP. A few doctors in the room stifled laughs,
but those in the immediate vicinity of the coat stared ahead, not
moving a muscle. Five minutes later, unable to contain my evil
twin... ZAP. The doctors who happened to be closest to the loud,
rude eruption wore a look of discomfort on their faces, as if to
say, "It wasn't I, dear esteemed stuffed coats!" It brought tears of
pure unadulterated joy to my eyes.

But is uncontrolled embarrassing painful gas, suffered by tens
of thousands in my town alone, many of whom ride in my elevator, a laughing matter? Of course it is!

But those whose internal GAS TANK is constantly on overdrive,
please take note.

Gas comes primarily from two sources. First, there are those
who swallow too much air. Some of the air-swallowers are the
worried; well, the nervous nellies who gulp air when anxious.
Others chew gum, eat too fast, or belch (belching actually causes
more air to be taken in).

Gas is also produced in the intestines by bacteria. In an honest-
to-goodness medical study, a twenty-eight-year-old man who had
a problem with "excess gas" meticulously recorded each toot for
three years. He changed his diets in order to determine the frequent flatulent factors. "Hey, Mom, remember you always wanted
me to contribute to medical research!" To no surprise, when
he went completely off carbohydrates, his gas problems ceased
almost altogether. In fact, to those patients who are concerned
about painful bloating and excessive gas, doctors advise stopping
carbohydrate ingestion. Stop dairy, broccoli, peas, beans, rad-
ishes, cabbage, brussels sprouts, and cauliflower. Stop apples, rai-
sins, prunes, and bananas. No fatty meats or fried foods. Avoid
carbonated beverages. Decrease fiber intake. One to two cap-
sules of peppermint three times a day might be helpful.

As for Louisa, her problem seemed to clear up when I went
on vacation.

SCRATCH AND LOSE

Prior to launching a herd of Boy Scouts out onto the world-famous Bowron Lake canoe circuit in beautiful British Columbia, we were briefed by the park ranger on a couple of the finer points of the circuit.

"First," barked the ranger, "have your bear stick ready at all times, and be prepared to use it properly."

"How exactly do we do that?" I inquired, purely for the benefit of the boys.

"Well," he replied, barely suppressing a smirk while reaching for a thick staff, "you take it like so, and then swing it like this into the knee of someone else in your group. Then you run like mad.

"Secondly," he begged, "please do not toss any food into the outhouse pits. Porcupines and bears will actually crawl down into the pits and we are none too pleased about being called out to fish some angry, smelly forest creature from the depths of a cesspool."

While the thought of having a burly black bear belching beneath your buttocks might be a tad disturbing, I'm not sure I'd like to be the next guy to use the commode after a perturbed porcupine was trapped beneath my keyster. "Hey, Bill, believe it or not, I think I picked up a few splinters sittin' in the honey-wagon. Got a light and some tweezers?"

What are some other pains in the butt that you as patients and we as doctors must deal with?

I would like to discuss three common anal ailments, which, to those of you in search of an interesting topic of conversation for your next date, will no doubt come as a blessing. Many mistakenly feel that symptoms of pain, bleeding, or itchiness are due to hemmorrhoids. Some patients have tried treating themselves, sometimes for years, with Preparation H or Absorbine Jr. or acupuncture when, had they simply seen a doctor, they could have been relieved of their misery long before.

1. Pruritus ani refers to a ferocious itch and irritation of the anal area. Despite all efforts to do otherwise, the urge to scratch or rub is so intense that it is difficult to resist even while sleeping. Pawing at one's derriere is not acceptable dinner etiquette (unless, of course, dinner is on the Bowron Lakes with a flock of Boy Scouts).

   This common and uncomfortable condition has been known to ruin promotions, distract fellow golfers, and spoil desserts. If you have this irritating affliction, do not suffer. See a doctor who will first make sure there is no pinworm or fungal skin infection. You will then be advised to avoid soaps and certain foods such as peppermint, caffeine, alcohol, and citrus. But most importantly, DO NOT SCRATCH! The itch-scratch cycle means that when skin is scratched, it releases chemicals, such as histamine, that invariably induce more itchiness. This leads to more scratching, hence the cycle. I treat this with a special salve combining an antibiotic, nitroglycerin paste (no explosion jokes here, please), and a bit of soothing steroid.

2. Anusitis refers to inflammation around the anal area and can be a cause of pruritus ani. The commonest of all anal problems, this inflammation leads to wetness, which in turn causes small cracks, infection, and itchiness. Like any inflamed joint or muscle, ice can be applied to reduce the swelling. If you find that scooping ice cubes out of your lemonade for this purpose is not terribly popular on your beach, you might consider purchasing a cryoprobe such as Anuice or Anurex (no kidding). Alternatively, try filling one finger of a rubber glove with water and freezing it. Smear the glove with Fucidin H cream and insert this probe twice a day for six minutes. Tremendous relief usually occurs within a couple of days. Ziplock the glove and place it in the freezer. (Warning: This might be a good time to teach your kids about the evils of stealing someone else's popsicles.)

3. Anal fissure means that the anus has a small, painful tear. Passing stool is akin to passing broken glass, and this condition, found

in kids and adults alike, is the commonest cause of painful rectal bleeding. Again, nitroglycerin is the key to treatment, as it
allows the tense sphincter to relax. Soften the stool with fiber,
water, and even medication. Should conservative treatment fail,
there is always a hungry surgeon more than eager to fix the face
of your fissures forever.

Finally, if that bummer of a pain happens to occur when
you're in the company of a bevy of Boy Scouts deep in the Canadian wilderness, don't forget to check... for quills.

I'D LIKE TO BUY A BOWEL

I like toilet paper. A nice, fluffy, soft, white-as-snow roll of joy. I
am fond of this puffy padded product of pillowy perfection not
only when camping in Giardia Springs National Park, but I also
like it perched pleasantly on the roll holder thingy in my bathroom. My dog, however, has determined that anything so spin-
ningly playful at her snout level must naturally be meant for her.
Daily and gaily she pops into the bathroom, grabs a quick porcelain drink, nabs the soft, white rolling toy of joy in her mouth,
performs a little rhythmic gymnastics unraveling piece after
piece, and when she's finished playing, eats it, sending it down
that puppy pipe of disaster to join other household snacks like
seventy-thousand-dollar shoes, leather couch, cat poop, etc.

And so, I've gone through a lot of toilet paper since getting a
dog. Though the cashier up at the local Piggly Wiggly doesn't
say anything as she scans seventy-one large bundles of Mr. Whip-
ple's TP, I know that she's thinking "IBS"—meaning, of course,
the "Idiot Bought Shreddies."

"Irritable Bowel Syndrome" is the diagnosis written on almost
half of all consults from gastroenterologists, who comment to
the GP in their reports that the most important thing to be done
is to "convince your patient that they haven't got anything more

sinister than IBS." Hey, if you've got it, it may not be sinister, but it's not exactly a picnic port-a-potty, either.

"Doctor, I have these awful cramps in my gut, and I know that colon cancer is pretty common these days," is not an uncommon fear expressed in my office by those who equate the severity of their discomfort with a severe diagnosis.

Since the mind and body are as intimately connected as Homer Simpson and honey crullers, stress can be worn physically in many ways. Those with twitchy skin get eczema; those with twitchy lungs, asthma; and those with twitchy hearts, rhythm disturbances. Others get twitchy headaches, but a whopping 10 to 15 per cent of the general population have IBS and so wear their stress in their bowels. Near exam time, university clinics are full of students who, despite their healthy diets of week-old triple-meat lover's/couch-lint pizza and Red Bull, develop abdominal cramping, bloating, diarrhea, or constipation. Similarly, athletes before big games, senators before audits, lawyers before... well, nothing really... I just thought a chapter on nasty bowel diseases should always have lawyers as honorable mentions.

Weddings are the worst for making a gut want to burst. Seventy-five per cent of those with IBS remain undiagnosed and so continue to suffer and worry. Thousands suffer on a daily basis, not realizing that there may be a simple remedy to their grief, but not wanting to see the doctor for fear of being told there is something evil up there, like cancer or Howard Stern. Others come armed with an Internet diagnosis: celiac disease, Crohn's, or alien abduction, but they're not yet willing to accept that it may just be a "twitchy bowel."

IBS has several subtypes, as I often explain to my dinner guests:

· IBS-C, whereby constipation is the prominent symptom;
· IBS-D, if diarrhea takes over during stress;
· IBS-A, if it alternates between diarrhea and constipation; and
· IBS-BS, if BS is involved.

The economic burden of IBS is only now coming to light. One interesting study shows that sufferers cost their employees $1,250 per year, to say nothing of the staff toilet paper supply . So getting properly diagnosed and treated not only means less pain and embarrassment, but more productivity and toilet paper, and for that . . . my dog thanks you.

GARFIELD AND THE CAT

In July 1881, U.S. president James Garfield was shot by a disgruntled (the gruntled ones were too busy gruntling) lawyer. Wanting to know if the bullet was going to send the president to that big Oval Office in the sky, doctors probed, poked, and prodded the wound with their unwashed fingers, until one finally poked too far and ruptured Garfield's liver. Still, the bullet could not be located.

Alexander Graham Bell, the famous inventor of graham crackers, was called in and asked to use his newfangled metal detector to find the leaded bullet. Bell had just tested his new device on Civil War vets' old injuries and was, each time, able to detect precisely where an old bullet lay. But as he waved his metal detector over the president, who would not take his eyes off the device for fear he was about to be electrocuted, the machine hummed as though the lead was everywhere! (Yes, he was a life-long politician.)

Incredulous at the outcome, Bell went home, honed his device, and tested it on a few more vets. One hundred per cent accurate. So back to the president he went, but once again—total body hum! Doctors went ahead and operated on the president, but in the wrong place altogether. No bullet. Poor old Garfield lay around this world for eighty days after he was shot, until the doctor-induced infections, liver ruptures, and hospital food killed him.

The bullet, it turned out, was lodged harmlessly in a cyst. It did not kill him. The over-meddling doctors did! Bell did not realize that he was up against another new invention that, at that time, had only been given to VIPS. President Garfield was convalescing on a brand-spanking-new coil-spring mattress. As the president lay on this metal bed frame, little did he realize that it would kill him by thwarting the only diagnostic testing of the time, metal detectors. Now you know. . . the rest of the story.

What a difference a century makes. Had Garfield had the good sense to have been shot one hundred years later, he would have been able to have a CAT scan (not Garfield the cat) or a PET scan (not that either), or even a simple X-ray. Doctors nowadays would either leave the bullet alone or remove it electively so that it could be auctioned off on eBay. Diagnostic equipment is advancing in leaps and bounds.

For example, were I to mention the word colonoscopy, many of you would immediately shred this book into kitty litter, dash off to the bedroom, toss a blanket over your head, curl up in the fetal position with your backside protectively planted against the wall, and rock to and fro. Certainly the thought of having a forty-six-foot serpentine (emphasis on the word serpent) tube inserted where no man or metal was ever meant to go gives most folks a serious case of the willies. But now comes virtual colonoscopy. What a virtual joy!

Colon cancer, the second most-common cancer killer in North America, begins as a wee polyp. Detected, it can easily be removed. Undiscovered, the polyp may grow to invade the bowel wall and kill its host. Most polyps are allowed to grow undetected due to the fact that most polyp-bearers avoid the very thought of a colonoscopoopy. Now, any significant polyp over a third of an inch can usually be found with a simple, non-invasive CAT scan. The scan takes all of ten minutes and can also detect other abdominal abnormalities including gallstones, aneurysms, and Jimmy Hoffa.

Slide the CAT scanner up an organ or two and now the amount of calcification in the coronary arteries can be assessed. Atherosclerotic plaques, i.e., Big Macs, Krispy Kremes, and jujubes congregate in the coronary arteries, where they then calcify. The radiologist can determine how much calcification plugs up your coronary arteries, then assign you a calcium score, which can determine your risk for having a heart attack. The more calcified, the more urgently a lifestyle should be altered to prevent heart attacks.

In court, the assassin/lawyer's (redundant?) actual defense was, "Guns don't kill presidents, doctors do." He was hanged.

The doctors had the gall to bill the Senate $85,000, which back in 1881 was enough to buy a senator's vote and tickets to the Rolling Stones. Instead, they were paid $10,000, made to publicly apologize, and then . . . audited.

ALL DUNG WITH DINNER

In my family, not having a TV has its pros and cons. While we spend less mind-numbing and obesity-inducing time with our noses glued to some senseless sitcom spew, some days we'd be thrilled to watch even the test pattern on channel 2. The boob tube has become a treat rather than a habit and so, whenever we have the occasion to watch TV, we sit spellbound, staring at commercials with slack-jawed intent as if watching the Queen of England belly dancing for a herd of Klingons.

And so it was that I found myself in a hotel room with my son watching with utter fascination a documentary on badgers. Were you aware, for example, that these resourceful excavators can sense where underground dungballs are hidden? What's a dungball? Well, if you'd watch more TV, you'd know! As any amateur dung beetleologist knows, dung beetles zip about collecting great wads of dung they then fashion into a large croquet-sized ball. As if rolling up a snowman, these dung beetles don wee scarves and go outside to frolic in the dung, making assorted dung angels, dung forts, and dungballs. But instead of sticking carrots or coal in the ball, they lay their larvae in it, assuming their progeny will be safe from any self-respecting animal with half a nose.

They didn't count on the disgusting badger. As we watched, the TV's larva-cam caught a badger clawing open a large ball of dung and then sticking its tongue into the center of it with great relish. As it slurped up a vile mix of large, juicy larvae and dung, I found it necessary to put down my pizza. In fact, I closed the box.

How could anything be interested in digging through such a nasty ball of poop? Yet we physicians, or at least lab techs, relish the opportunity to do much the same, usually minus the tongue and larvae.

The most sought-after information in a stool specimen is the presence of hidden blood. Last year 60,000 North Americans died of a largely preventable disease, colorectal cancer (CRC). Another 150,000 got the news that they have contracted this second deadliest of all cancers, lung cancer being the first.

If you are a non-smoker, CRC is the cancer most likely to do you in. The good news: CRC is generally a slow-growing beast that gives hints that it is about to turn nasty by leaking very small amounts of blood into the stool. CRC begins its life as an easily removable polyp. While most colonic polyps are small and pose no threat, larger polyps, which take five to ten years to grow, are precursors to cancer.

For this reason, every man, woman, and child over age fifty should have an annual fecal occult blood test (FOBT). See a doctor, who will give you three test cards to take home. Consume a high-fiber diet for two days, avoiding broccoli, cauliflower, Vitamin C, and red meat, all of which can affect the test reagents. On three separate days, take a small stick and (retch, gag) apply stool to these cards, then fold them back up. These cards look like scratch and wins, but please advise the kids or any lotto players in the house that should they open the card and enthusiastically rub, they would only scratch and lose.

Discard the stick far away from coffee stir sticks. Return the card lovingly to your doctor accompanied by a note of appreciation for what he has to go through just to ensure your good health. Alternatively, to the chagrin of the Cliff Clavins of the world, you can mail the sample in, hoping the postman's pet badger doesn't accompany him on his route.

Through the miracle of modern medical magic, the doctor can instantly detect the presence of blood in the stool. While blood does not always mean cancer, it does mean that further investigation, in the form of a colonoscopy or CT colonography, is warranted.

As screening tests go, FOBT has proven to save lives through early detection of a cancer that is usually not bothersome to its victim until it has spread ominously beyond the bowel wall. Since 1984, death by CRC has decreased by 2 per cent per year, due to enhanced screening and better mail service.

So please, screen yourself. Though it may sound less than palatable, go and see your doctor and have this simple test done. In addition to keeping us all humble, it may save your life. Please don't make us badger you.

HIS, HERS,

( )

and THEIRS

• • •

HIS AND HERS

Along with his and her towels, his and her cars, his and her razors, and his and her negligees, please add his and her cancers. The prostate and the breast, both capable of harboring hormone-sensitive cancers, possess some intriguing similarities.

At birth, the prostate gland is about the size of a pea, while a newborn brain is the size of a ripe avocado. By adulthood, the prostate resembles the avocado, while the male brain (as I'm repeatedly reminded by numerous females in my life) tends to resemble the pea.

The prostate's job is to provide a fluid that nourishes sperm. Eighteen nanoseconds after nourishment, the well-fed sperm cheerfully heads off to work on an egg hunt, never to return. The breast's job is to provide a fluid that nourishes children. Eighteen years later, the well-nourished child will reluctantly be egged on to find work, always to return.

Stats
Perhaps the most unfortunate similarity between the breast and the prostate is the fact that, this year, 200,000 women and

200,000 men in North America will be diagnosed with breast and prostate cancers respectively. Of these, 44,000 women will succumb to their disease, while 37,000 men with prostate cancer will not survive. Prostate cancer is now the most commonly diagnosed cancer in men. It is the second leading cause of cancer death in males, trailing only lung cancer for that dubious distinction. Breast cancer is the most commonly diagnosed cancer in women. One woman in eight will develop breast cancer in her lifetime. Both cancers can be made more aggressive by our so-called sex hormones. Testosterone can speed up the spread of prostate cancer, and estrogen worsens some breast cancers. Both cancers are more apt to occur in relatives of those who have had them. Oddly, both prostate and breast cancers are rare in Japan.

Clinical Presentation
Both cancers present with PAINLESS lumps in their respective gland. When a woman comes in to the office with a sore breast, my first job is to reassure her that breast cancer generally is not painful until the very later stages. Most painful breast lumps are cysts or teeth left by a weaning child. Similarly, when a man presents to the office stating his prostate is sore, my first job is to reassure him that he probably has no idea where his prostate is.

Diagnosis
Here the similarities tend to diverge. Women are encouraged to conduct breast self-exams (BSEs). Rubber gloves are not necessary. A prostate self-exam, in contrast, tends to be a tad awkward and is frowned upon in most social circles. A prostate exam, called a DRE (digital rectal exam), should be performed only by a trained professional. Attempt this at home and even your dog will likely run away. Current recommendations are for men to have an annual DRE after the age of forty-five.

The breast self-exam should be performed monthly, about a week after a woman's period. The best method for BSE involves moving the fingers up and down rapidly on the breast while moving the hand up and down the breast. This is called the lawnmower.

Men could also attempt the lawnmower, but only on lawns.

After age forty, a woman should have a screening mammogram every one to two years and annually after the age of fifty. The mammogram is a diagnostic test wherein the breast is placed between two paddles and squeezed and squished flat.

Realizing that this story focuses on similarities between prostates and breasts, most men, by now, have recoiled in horror, tossing the book across the room should any comparable test exist for the prostate. Fear not, brave lads; the prostate will not be squished flat in any machine. Instead, if a suspicious prostate lump is detected on a DRE, a really sharp needle is jammed into the prostate, and a piece of it is torn out for a biopsy. Feel better?

CAUSE FOR PAUSE

One of the great misnomers in the English language is the term "menopause," which, of course, has nothing to do with men—other than the fact that during this phase of a woman's life, men tend to pause in fear every time they hear the kitchen knife drawer open. Men, too, have a change of life, called andropause. It isn't as dramatic as menopause, when a woman may go to bed one night reciting Gandhi and awake the next morning scrawling phrases from *Helter Skelter* in lipstick on the bathroom mirror. Rather, andropause is a more gradual change of life regulated by the incremental loss of testosterone.

"Andro" comes from the fact that most men are on an emotional par with androids and the "pause" from the break they take from being real men as they start whining like Chewbacca. This would almost be bearable if the andropausians could also inherit some of Chewie's hair. Andropausoid hair tends to get confused and, not unlike its owners, forgets to ask for directions and grows inwardly from the scalp, emerging daintily from the nose, ears, and eyebrows.

From about age thirty, men begin to lose their testosterone at a rate of about 1 to 2 per cent per year. This means that, should they ever live to ninety-two years of age, they will have zero testosterone left and could thus either play for the New York Rangers or sing falsetto for the Beach Boys. Some athletes, however, have been known to mysteriously *gain* 1 to 2 per cent testosterone per year (by needle) so that by the time *they* are ninety-two, they have bad acne and are challenging George Foreman between stints as an NFL tackle. For a man to replenish his hormone levels, he can either stand downwind of Barry Bonds or see his youthful doctor, who is actually eighty-six years old but has known the secret for years.

The doctor, in turn, may diagnose a condition actually known as ADAM (Androgen Decline in Aging Men). This may make the man feel on par with his wife, who last week could've been diagnosed with EVE (Emitting Violent Estrogens).

The symptoms of an andropausal man include a decrease in energy, strength, happiness, libido, sleep, memory, and body hair, and an increase in weight, moodiness, wakefulness, and hot flashes. Yes, hot flashes.

Testosterone Physiology 101:

1. As a male ages, he produces less of the sleep hormone melatonin (not effectively replaced by melatonin pills); therefore, he
2. Gets less deep sleep, which is the time that the testes enjoy making testosterone
3. Which he now makes less of. Conversely, he makes more leptin instead, a hormone found in fat cells, so subsequently he gains
4. More fat, less energy. Weight up, happiness down.

Baby boomers refuse to grow old gracefully as they continue to redefine the passages of life. Over the hill is no longer thirty but rather when the grandkids are thirty. Octogenarians can be found requesting tie-dyed Depends, Elton John corrective lenses, and Scary Spice orthopedic shoes. So why not hormones? Our bodies were simply not intended to outlive our hormones. We were supposed to live to fifty and then die or move to Florida. But now, like track stars, men are replacing dwindling testosterone levels by means of a pill, a shot, or even a gel. Though they haven't grown from 5'4" to 5'14" or become raving stallions, they have become more robust, more vigorous, and even happier.

And now, just the very act of buying the medicine can apparently boost testosterone levels. From the Most Unlikely Merger file, a pharmacy in my neighborhood has actually combined with a hardware store. Apparently, when you purchase a month's supply of testosterone, you get 40 per cent off a cordless rechargeable power drill. Coincidence?

ORCHIDS BY THE PAIR

Should you possess a deep and fervent passion for orchids, I strongly suggest that you stop reading this article and turn from this page to something more edifying, like the back cover. For those still reading, you are about to learn some real medical terms that might affect the way you look at orchids. Unfortunately for flower lovers, the root of an orchid happens to resemble the male testicle. Greek doctors thought it would be cool to name various organs after various plants. "Xerxes, cut along the patient's creeping myrtle until you reach the petunia, then reach in and remove the honeysuckle." And so, to this day, any medical term that deals with the male nether region employs the term "orchid." For example:

- Orchitis—inflammation of the testes, often caused by mumps.
- Orchiectomy—surgical removal of a testicle (usually as a result of cancer).
- Cryptorchidism—when a newborn's testicle has not descended from the abdomen down into its "vase."
- Orchiopexy—the procedure of repairing cryptorchidism by retrieving the testicle and stitching it to the scrotum.

By now, most men reading this are wincing and grimacing and have both hands tucked protectively between their clenched knees. I am now typing with my nose. But how often have you guys caught yourself admitting that you'd give your left orchid to be the world's greatest athlete? Lance Armstrong, arguably the world's best athlete, and possibly its most inspirational one, did just that in 1996. Ranked the world's top cyclist, Lance was diagnosed with an advanced testicular cancer that had spread to his brain and lungs. Critically ill, his chance of survival was less than 50 per cent. His French sponsor, knowing the odds, pulled out. Lance underwent an orchiectomy and time-trialed new and aggressive chemotherapy. He beat the odds, beat the cancer, and went on to beat the top cyclists in the world! And he did so with panache. Not only did he re-enter the grueling cycling circuit, he went on to win the prestigious Tour de France seven consecutive years from 1999 to 2005. During this amazing feat, he emphatically stamped his victory over testicular cancer when his wife gave birth to twin girls. One good orchid produced two more-kids.

When paranoid medical students are first taught how to check for certain diseases, they often examine their own bodies first. For example, when our professor discussed lymph nodes, the entire class would, in unison, begin palpating our own necks or the necks of those nearby. For the next week we were all pawing, probing, and prodding for lymphomas or other nodal disasters. So when we were taught that the commonest cancer of men age fifteen to thirty-five is testicular cancer, well, the sight that followed was not a pretty one. A full third of us ended up concerned, if not convinced, that we were about to donate an orchid to the great flowerpot in the sky.

Testicular cancer is usually not terribly deadly, and in fact, not all that common. However, the incidence of testicular cancer has risen 51 per cent in the past forty years. Oddly enough, cryptorchidism (see above), a well-known risk factor for testicular cancer, has risen 60 per cent over the same time frame. Another oddity is that testicular cancer attacks white men almost exclusively. Maybe this is why we can't jump.

So current recommendations are that once a month, males over age fifteen should do a careful orchid inspection, best done in a warm shower. Cancer will feel like a hard, painless peanut. If cancer is present, then orchiectomy is the definitive cure. For those concerned about how things will look at the beach after an orchiectomy, silicone and now saline prostheses are available. If you think that's nuts (sorry), then you'll love the fact that even male dogs can have replacements (called "Neuticles") after they have been fixed. Makes us all feel a little more confident around the hydrant.

HAGGIS HERNIA

Went to a Scottish Highland Games in that grand duchy of Scotland known as Enumclaw, Washington. Easy to spot the Scottish festival by the excessively long ticket lines created by heated negotiations of the entrance fee by each and every patron. Lasses and laddies pranced and flinged about on their delicate wee toes, real men sported kilts, real women and a fellow named Gordon sported "Official Kilt Inspector" T-shirts. Gathering of the clans, eating of the official oatmeal, parading of the dogs, blaring of the pipes and drums (named after the parts of the lungs and ears that no longer function as God meant them to in those who use such instruments).

The games portion included tossing the haggis, the hammer throw, and the intriguing caber toss. A caber looks like a telephone pole on steroids, much, I suspect, like those who toss them. They lift the caber up, try to balance it, and then, with a mighty heave that would make Robert the Bruce pop his porridge, toss the caber up in the air and hope it lands on the opposite end and then falls over on one of the other competitors.

Now, what others didn't notice but I did, being the consummate medical professional, was the hernias that these caber tossers were experiencing, judging by the sudden inflation of the front of their kilts as they grimaced and clutched their wee sporrans.

Hernias were/are the bread and butter of surgeons, or at least the bread part, as they make a lot of it fixing weekend caber tossers. Hernias come in all sizes and sorts and can involve places like the stomach, the groin, and of course, the attractive belly-button bulge. A hernia is simply a weakness of a wall that allows something behind it to squeeze out partway: a piece of fat, a piece of bowel, Sigourney Weaver. Twenty million groin (inguinal) hernias are repaired each year worldwide. Pregnancy, age, and the widening of the waistline can lead to the weakening of supportive muscles, thus allowing hernias to... well... herniate.

Males get more hernias than females by seven to one, usually while operating the freakin' dill pickle jar or playing pickup cabers in the backyard. The main problem with hernia bulges, besides ruining your Lululemons, is that a piece of bowel can get caught in the hernia and twist on itself or get pinched off, conditions known as strangulation and incarceration (sort of what happened to my Uncle Jake). Heal-with-steel surgeons earn their bread and butter with hernia repairs, but occasionally, patients may suffer some post-operative pain that can last for months. Some doctors feel all hernias should be fixed before they get larger and harder to repair, others only if they cause discomfort.

In children, all groin hernias should be considered for surgical repair, but the umbilical (navel) outies never need to be fixed before the age of two. By age five, if they still have a large outie, then they might need a repair, as the psychological scar of having classmates using their belly button to play horseshoes will last at least until snacktime. Many adults with umbilical hernias like to get them fixed so they can waddle right back onto the beach, swinging those love handles to and fro with abandon.

Most hernias are fixed with a strong mesh device that doubles as a broccoli filter. It should stay strong and in fact is guaranteed to stay fixed, though the warranty is void should you... travel to Scotland.

OLD GROINS AND IMMATURE MEN

I enjoy few things more than playing hockey. Actually, I'm a little deeper than that. I also enjoy watching hockey, table hockey, roller hockey, playing hooky, Stompin' Tom, hockey gear, hockey pools, and Jell-O. But I, like many of you, am not as young as I was a year ago. This means that in order to win, I must now resort to wilier tactics, such as tripping, slashing, blaming others, and reminding the ref that he may one day find himself lying naked on my examining table.

But for a few moments last week, I thought I was twenty-one again. I accelerated on the ice—like really, really fast, dude. My groin was not happy about this twenty-one-year-old thing. It groaned, whined, roared, and then snapped. A few more strides and I was toast. A groin pull/strain/tear/owwie.

Reacting in typical hockey macho style, I tossed my helmet, broke my stick over Scottie's head, and lay on the ice making snow angels, or at least half a snow angel. I writhed and grimaced and clutched myself so dramatically that soccer scouts started salivating. The next morning I prepared to ooze out of bed, but my groin was still in the penalty box. Unable to move my left leg, I logrolled onto my stomach, pivoted about my navel axis, arched my back, and slid off the mattress backward, like a confused walrus.

Now, as much as the condition of my groin is, no doubt, of great concern to you, this is about physiotherapy, not the state of my groin. (That story will be told in my next book, entitled *Dr. Dave, A Real Groiner,* soon to be made into a TV docudrama featuring George Clooney as myself, with groin stunts and clutches performed by Michael Jackson and Manchester United.)

Recalling a painful teenage experience with Absorbine Jr. and a previous groin strain, I decided that, instead of self-medicating, I would visit my local physiotherapist. Physiotherapy is not something doctors necessarily know a whole lot about. We are the diagnosers; they are the fixer-uppers. If a patient limps into the office, holding a kneecap in their hands, we diagnose "sore leg," prescribe them a drug to make us feel complete, and send them to physio to get fixed up.

As I lay on the physio's table, Barb (perfect name) marched in towing an ultrasound machine. Now, u/s is an excellent treatment modality, though I must admit I was a tad leery of anything attached to an electrical outlet getting that close to my nether regions. But my groin pain was growing pain, so I let the machine do its thing. Ultrasound not only decreases inflammation but also speeds up healing by allowing the muscle fibers to properly align. In addition, therapeutic u/s has been shown to expedite fracture healing. And I was amazed! After a few minutes, I was all but able to throw away my crutches and hop out of the office, which I did with such glee that I tripped and pulled my groin. So I returned the next day, wanting to know what other instruments these physios employ to heal foolishly injured patients.

"What other instruments do you employ to heal foolishly injured patients?" I asked.

"Well," replied Barb, "we have interferential, an electrical suction-cup device that relieves pain and stimulates muscle, causing it to contract and relax."

"To be used when?" I gasped, as I reflexively guarded my injury with a magazine.

"When muscles need to be strengthened, such as after a joint, muscle, or bone injury or operation. It can also be used to strengthen intrinsic back muscles, allowing those with back pain to rebalance their spines. And over here we have a traction device"—she pointed to a device with a pulley, chains, a dial, and MORE WIRES CONNECTED TO AN OUTLET!—"commonly known as 'the rack.' Assorted back and neck pains can benefit from traction."

"Hence the term 'physioterrorist'."

"But our greatest tools are these," she remarked as she reached into her pocket and pulled out a vicious pair of hands, conveniently attached to a muscular pair of arms. To make matters worse, they smelled like... Absorbine Jr. (For the final outcome of this groin therapy, please see the movie, or read chapter 11 of my next book, entitled "It's Just a Little Limp!")

PUMPED-UP PROSTATES

"Okay, Bloggins, we'll check out that ol' prostate of yours today."

"Ahh..." gulps Bloggins, "how so, doc?"

"Well, let's just say we'll use digital technology. Now bend over and smile."

The prostate check is the most hated of all medical tests (by patients as well).

This one is for men with prostates and the women who love them (the men). Prostate, an odd word, was always tough for me to differentiate from *prostrate*, as I could never recall which one, when ill, rendered you the other.

The prostate is a walnut-sized and -shaped gland that sits at the base of the bladder. It is not much smarter than the average walnut, and only slightly more active. It wakes up only for sex; otherwise, it just lies there prostrate and thinks about... well... probably not much more than sex. Rarely does it ponder politics, the Stanley Cup play-offs, or why it lives so close to a bladder. All it thinks about is sex; this, in fact, is its sole purpose for living.

The prostate is the Arnold Schwartznegger of the male reproductive system. After forty-five years or so of contemplating sex and doing steroids (testosterone), the prostate gets bulked up pretty good. It gets mean and pumped, and, as it enlarges, it begins to strangle the outlet pipe of the bladder (the urethra).

Prostatic enlargement occurs in all men to a degree, but when it buffs up to the point of really putting the squeeze on the poor urethra, well, you got yerself a bonafide, brag-at-the-rink, whine-to-the-missus male disease medical condition called BPH. "Geez, Art, I know I should've scored there, but I got BPH." The whole team will offer guesses as to what this means, ranging from Belches Per Hour to Bad Perm Hairdo to Bulging Purple Hemmorrhoids. You will stand and declare, "Nope, I got Benign Prostatic Hypertrophy," putting the emphasis on *benign*. This is *not* cancer.

How can you tell if you are one of the 20 per cent of men over age fifty with this condition?

1. First you must be male; women do not have prostates. The only time women are bothered by prostates is when Mr. Bloggins is up five times a night, making a point of telling Mrs. B that his prostate has "flared again."
2. Frequency—going all the time, especially at night when you may be up five or six times.
3. Difficulty stopping and starting—having rushed out of bed with that urge to void, you stand and stand and stand and can usually whistle the entire soundtrack of *Oklahoma!* before anything actually works. Once started, you may only dribble, and then, just as you think you're done—whoops—you're halfway through *Phantom of The Opera* before you finally zip up.
4. Yer yerinary stream weakens. No longer are you able to write your name in the snow (braggarts could also do their middle name and add a nickname at the end). With BPH you'd be lucky to dot the i's and cross the t's.
5. Inability to delay, or urgency. You know every washroom at the mall intimately but, should the stall be occupied by someone whistling the complete works of Andrew Lloyd Webber, you may get...
6. Incontinence—occurs even in Antarctica.

Up until recently, the only way to remedy BPH was by a roto-rooter procedure called a TURP (transurethral resection of the prostate), in which bits and pieces of the gland are chopped out through the urethra. Though it is the second most-common operation in men over age sixty-five, it is not without its problems. More recently, two kinds of drugs that really help have come "down the pipe." One prevents Arnold from actually getting its steroids but takes a while to work. Another tells Arnold to relax those muscles and let the poor urethra go. And now some new procedures are available, one involving laser and another in which a small antenna is passed into the urethra and microwaves are pulsed in that burn the prostate. Though this is an expensive procedure, side benefits include coming home after the procedure full of microwaves, pointing your prostate at the frozen chicken, and having it cooked in eight minutes.

ALL JUICE, NO SEEDS

The military has an odd knack of referring to any nerve-racking medical procedure as a "parade," as though the thought of a marching band, twirling batons, and juggling politicians in clown suits lessens the inevitable discomfort. "Needle parade," for example, is the lining up of the troops for inoculations. My personal favorite was "Vas parade" when, every Friday morning, all those "wishing" vasectomies would present to the clinic. "The Colonel is here about his Privates," the Medical Assistant would announce gleefully as he marched the shaking officer into the OR. Upon completion of the procedure, the Med A would turn to the vulnerable, vibrating, vasectomized victim and hand him a glass of orange juice.

"Welcome to the club, sir."

"What club?"

"The Sunkist orange club—all juice and no seeds."

PARENTAL DEBATES between husbands and wives include who should change the diapers, who gets up at night with the baby, who goes to Billy's first violin lesson, who meets Billy's angry principal, who tells Billy about the facts of life, and finally, when no more Billys are desired, who gets fixed.

Vasectomy or tubal ligation. The male or the female. The woman or the wimp.

I hope to solve this debate here, and my final recommendations will be based purely on the medical facts, with a slight bias toward those from whom I get tickets to the NHL All-Star game.

The vas deferens are the tubes that men possess that transport Billy's future sibs. They must be cut and tied off if this is to no longer occur. (An old doctorly joke: there is a vas deferens between a man and a woman.)

More than 600,000 vasectomies are performed annually in North America, with the newest improvement on the procedure being the no-scalpel vasectomy (NSV). While this may conjure up images of a surgeon using assorted dental instruments or really sharp fingernails, in fact, the procedure is done through a very small puncture in the scrotum. NSV is done under local anesthetic with what the surgeon will describe as just a "small mosquito bite." Small or not, to most men, a needle in that part of the anatomy may as well be the freakin' Jaws of Life. Routine mosquito bites become vicious saber-tooth attacks.

No-scalpel vasectomy involves no stitches, no shaving, no scalpel, and no sniveling. Advantages of this procedure include less bleeding, less infection, and less time someone is fiddling with their nether regions. The vas is severed and the tubes are tied off. There is no decrease in libido, and the failure rate— failure meaning Billy gets a sister—is less than 1 per cent. Sometimes a little lump can develop at the site, but except for some occasional post-op swelling, few complications result.

It must be considered a permanent sterilization. Reversal is expensive and not terribly successful; it's like trying to take two strands of thread and align the ends precisely head to head, then sewing them together.

Tubal ligations require penetration to the abdominal cavity. The fallopian tubes leading from the ovaries to the uterus are clipped, cauterized, or cut. Again, it is a relatively simple procedure with few complications. Done right after childbirth, this is easy and effective (and the patient is usually highly motivated). Though this, too, must be considered permanent, reversal is somewhat more successful than with vasectomies.

The vasectomy is safer, easier, and quicker. The disadvantages are that it is not as easily reversible, and it has to be performed on... wimps.

COMB-FREE LIVING

"If you don't have it, flaunt it."—Mr. Reynolds

Mr. Reynolds was an unusual and frightening physics teacher. I was enrolled in his high school class, Unusual and Frightening Physics 101. To teach us the finer principles of physics, he would bring in radioactive material for us to play with, boil plastic flamingos, and even shoot off a gun (long before it was routine recess recreation).

But what made him even more unusual was that he was completely bald. Not a speck of hair on his twenty-nine-year-old head, eyelashes included. Made Yul Brenner look like a hippie. Compared to Mr. Reynolds, Kojak was a Chia Pet. Think Yoda. It was as though some experiment involving liquid nitrogen and Nair had gone wrong. Though I loved his class, I lost my composure one day when he brought in a bowling ball to demonstrate inertia and friction. It sent me into a massive giggling spasm, the type where, to keep from blurting out, you bite the inside of your cheek so hard you bleed.

"What's so funny, Hepburn?" Mr. Reynolds asked.

"Well, to be honest, sir, I was just picturing your eyeglasses on that ball and..."

Later that day, while in detention, I finally screwed up the courage to ask, "Sir, how did you get to be so bald?"

"Well," he responded with a sigh, "I was a hairy guy once, then suddenly, POOF, it was gone, in one week. The doctor called it alopecia areata totalis. I call it the solar panel to my brain."

Alopecia areata

One day out of the blue, your immune system, like your parents, might get sick and tired of your hairdo. It will attack the hair follicles and suddenly, over a period of one to two weeks, round bald patches will develop over the scalp. While this usually resolves spontaneously in three to six months, sometimes these bald patches coalesce, like that freaky mercurial cop in *Terminator* that just would not die. The patches can merge to the point that the entire head becomes bare, a condition called alopecia totalis. Sometimes, as in the case of Mr. Reynolds, the immune system takes out all body hair, including eyelashes and facial hair. I recall a patient who had this same alopecia universalis at age sixteen, only to have all of her hair suddenly grow back at age forty-one! "Honey, do you remember where I put that Lady Gillette thing?"

Male-pattern baldness

Roughly 50 per cent of men will develop a "really wide part," often decorated by three exceedingly long hairs stretched across the scalp for warmth. These Friar Tucks of hairdom usually hail from families with a genetic predisposition to baldness. Even women from families with a history heavy in chrome domes may develop male-pattern baldness. Like most of the world's problems, we can blame this comb-free living on testosterone. Genetics determine how much testosterone will be converted to its nastier form, DHEAS, in hair follicles. Testosterone and hair follicles don't get along. Testosterone, being tougher, wins.

Men who are eunuchs or who have had their testicles

removed for other reasons (see Clinton) *stop* losing their hair! Hey, some guys hate being bald. While most of North America's 80 million balding men just say no to drugs, rugs, and plugs, the rest spend a slick 7 billion dollars a year on hair loss treatment. One drug, finasteride, taken orally, will prevent testosterone from torturing hair follicles. Minoxidil lotion also helps to reseed the recede, though it must be taken continually, as hair loss resumes when the medication is stopped.

Trichotillomania

The deliberate, compulsive pulling out of one's own hair is a bizarre yet fairly common cause of unexplained bald spots. This may range from mild twisting and yanking of a few strands to a more severe grabbing and hauling out of massive clumps. Before age six it is primarily boys who engage in such behavior, often perfecting this talent by practicing on their sisters. After age six, girl trichotillomaniacs outnumber boys ten to one. Treatment involves medications to treat compulsive behavior disorders or else cutting off the hair completely—which may seem harsh but hey, it beats what has to get cut off to treat male-pattern baldness.

HIBERNATING HAIR

"Doc, I'm losing my hair, and I'm not happy about it."

"Yep, you're certainly pretty sparse up on the old noodle wagon. Not a problem, the women love it, kind of a testosterone billboard on your head."

"Umm, I *am* a woman."

"Ah. Well, in that case, you have a problem."

"Can you make my hair come back?"

"Well, I can't pull hares out of a hat. But did you happen to notice anything different in your life about three months ago?"

"Can't think of anything. I'd ask my husband, but he's at home with the baby."

"And how old is the baby?"

"Three months old, bright as a button."

"Really? Adopted?"

"Not that I know of. But I wish we had adopted. The birth was awful, and I ended up having a C-section. I almost didn't make it. Bert was already checking the policies but I pulled through, thanks to his motivating words: 'Clarisse, don't worry, if you don't make it, they'll pay within ninety days.' Then, after the birth, my thyroid gland went wonky."

"Did you lose a lot of weight after the birth?"

"Not really. I'm down about eighty pounds, nothing noticeable yet."

THE NORMAL HUMAN scalp is a forest of 100,000 hairs, which is roughly equivalent to the amount that my hirsute hound, Sasquatch, sheds onto the kitchen floor every day.

The cells at the base of a hair follicle divide every twelve hours, allowing hair to grow a quarter of an inch per month. This growing hair, called the anagen hair, will grow for several months or years, depending on our genes and the mood of our barber. Finally, the exhausted cells in the hair follicle shut down. The hair no longer grows, but becomes a resting hair called a telogen hair. After about three months, this telogen hair decides to retire completely from the scalp. It buys a Winnebago and some ugly shorts and heads to Palm Someplace. We shed fifty to seventy-five telogen hairs per day. After a telogen hair departs, a fresh anagen hair takes its place. At any one time, the average human head houses 90 per cent anagen hairs, 9 per cent telogen, and 1 per cent lice.

But these anagen hairs are a sensitive lot and are easily insulted. An insult can be in the form of rapid weight loss, acute illnesses with high fevers, iron deficiency, childbirth, thyroid problems, surgery, and medications like hormones, beta blockers, and even aspirin. When they get upset, many of these anagen hairs shut down their follicle cells, call it quits, and become a telogen hair. Three months later they do the typical telogen thing and leave the scalp en masse, a condition known as telogen effluvium. Shedding of more than one hundred hairs per day ensues, and though telogen effluvium may begin abruptly, it might continue for several years. Telogen effluvium occurs primarily in women. Though surgery, childbirth, and weight loss can be precipitants, the cause of telogen effluvium, like women themselves, remains a mystery for the most part (no pun intended). Though the hair often grows back, it may remain thin. There is no specific treatment other than treating the underlying cause (i.e., correcting the iron or thyroid problem, replacing a medication, or reversing the childbirth).

Telogen effluvium is also responsible for a bizarre medical condition called toe tourniquet syndrome. New mothers have some degree of telogen effluvium three to four months after giving birth. If their hair is long, it may fall into the crib and surreptitiously become entangled in the baby's toes or fingers. This hair acts like a tourniquet by painfully cutting off the circulation of the extremity, occasionally leading to amputation of the digit.

So, molting mothers, if your head is bare, please be aware: your baby's crying may be due to your hair.

FATAL ATTRACTIONS

Ever seen a fish fish? No no? Well, say hello to the anglerfish, a disgusting-looking denizen of the deep that actually fishes for other fish. A fishing rod hangs off her head and emits a little light to attract supper, not unlike the way my Uncle Ernie hunts and fishes. But the light also attracts a potential mate who, unable to see well deep in the ocean, is drawn to the light. Upon realizing it is a female, he sinks his teeth into her and is her mate for life. Even if the light gets bright and he actually gets a peek at his repulsive bride, it's too late for cold fins; they are wed until shark do them part.

The anglerfish was part of a museum exhibit entitled "Fatal Attractions," showing instances of dangerous mating behaviors of creatures of the wild, including bugs, fish, confused moose, a rather obscene snail and his love dart, Michael Douglas, etc.

The male octopus, a known cannibal, will either mate or eat'm the meat (spot all three anagrams?). A male grouse has to expose himself (so to speak) in an open area in order to properly show off his plumage, but this also attracts predators that give him plenty to grouse about. The mandrill, not unlike Barbara, caught my eyes as this baboon-like creature with the brilliant blue, red, and gold face also develops the same colors in his butt and genitals in order to appear more attractive. ("Oooh, Betty, is that the southbound end of a northbound mandrill, or the north-bound end of a . . . oh, who cares, he's HOT!") The male hobo spider shakes what his momma gave him, and if he dances well, then she has him over for dinner and they mate; if he dances poorly she just has him for dinner. Come across a spider prac-ticing the eight-legged macarena, leave the poor guy alone—his evening/life depends on it.

"I'm gonna kill him" is the usual response of those who have discovered that their liaison of love has left them with skin sores or a baggage of bumps. Yes, I am talking about the all-too-common experience doctors undergo of telling a patient that they have herpes.

HERPES SIMPLEX is the virus responsible for cold sores of the face and hot sores of the nether regions. A patient's worst fears are too often followed by a patient's burst tears as the diagnosis of herpes is explained to them. They often then deeply desire to bring a fatal conclusion to that attractive source of their disease.

Sixty million adults in North America have genital herpes. This is the same number as there are Yankees fans, which is why one should never cheer for the Yankees. One in five adults has genital herpes. While this could lead to an interesting dinner-party guessing game or an office pool ("I'll put twenty dollars on Ralph, Frank, and Loretta"), the numbers are changing precipitously. There are 1 million new infections served every year. For overall prevalence, genital herpes infects more people than all other sexually transmitted infections combined. The problem is that 90 per cent of those who have genital herpes don't know it. Most actually only find out after someone they have been with contracts symptomatic herpes... from them. This little devastation in the life of that patient begins in my office. Well... umm... not the infection part, usually. The vast majority of transmissions of this highly infectious virus come from asymptomatic carriers who honestly haven't got a clue.

When it does become symptomatic, it may range from painful sores known as ulcers to small fissures (cracks in the skin), or even burning on urination. But the misconception that folks have to have something that hurts in order for it to be herpes really isn't the case. Besides the obvious unpleasantness, herpes can be extremely dangerous and even fatal to a newborn as it passes through an infected birth canal. So unless you want to cheer for the Yankees... be careful what you fish for.

DR. PAP AND PALS

"I'm sorry to tell you this, Miss Bloggins, but you have a nasty case of genital warts."

"Noooo, not warts! I'd rather have cancer!"

"Well, I'm afraid you might have that, too."

Unfortunately human papilloma virus (HPV) is responsible for both unsightly genital warts (and most of the sightly ones) *and* cervical cancer, one of the most devastating diseases of womankind. In 1935 George Papanicolaou ("Pap" to his buddies) of Cornell University discovered that by taking a wee scraping from the opening to the womb, he was able to determine, under a microscope, if pre-cancerous cells were brewing. Little did Dr. Pap know that he was looking for damage caused by the human papilloma virus ("Pap" to its viral buddies). Papillomas for Doctor Papanicolaou. Pap looking for pap (not related, apparently). Poor George eventually became so disenchanted with having the Pap test named after him that he left science and became an annoying celebrity photographer, only later to discover they were called . . . paparazzi.

Consider these sobering facts:

- In 2004, fourteen North American women died of cervical cancer each day.
- Eighty-five per cent of them had not had routine Papanicolaou smears.
- Every two and a half minutes, a woman on this planet dies of cervical cancer.
- As a result of lack of screening facilities, cervical cancer is the leading cause of cancer death in women in third-world countries.
- Fifteen thousand North American women will be diagnosed with cervical cancer this year.
- A turtle can actually breathe through its butt, right past its prostate.

The main purpose of Mr. Papanicolaou's test is to detect the presence of HPV-induced pre-cancerous lesions. The Pap screening test is the reason that cervical cancer has gone from being the most-common deadly cancer of women to a cancer so low in North America that only five thousand women die of cervical cancer each year (most of whom have not had recent Pap smears). But Pap smears, de test that women detest, may soon be a thing of de past.

In the exciting world of tumor immunotherapeutics (exciting because you can impress your friends and score huge Scrabble points with jargon like that), an HPV vaccine is available that prevents cervical cancer and warts! A vaccine for cancer. It is geared toward the junior-high-school-aged girls before they become sexually active, which is, like, totally awesome. Sixty per cent of women contract HPV within five years of beginning sexual activity. Unfortunately, HPV can have a deadly consequence. Nuns do not get cervical cancer or genital warts (a "pap"al state?), though Sister Mary Mashbone from my school used to have a wart on her chin that looked like it would give you cancer, a stroke, and several heart attacks if it ever touched you.

Other vaccines are currently being developed against assorted cancers such as ovarian and breast cancer. And for the prostatic man in your life, work is being done on a vaccine against prostate cancer, which should make all men who hate prostate checks ecstatic, and, of course, allow turtles to breathe a little easier.

BESTEST BABIES

"Hi, Mom, it's your favorite son."

"Bill?"

"Good one, Mom."

"Susan?"

"No."

"Well, that leaves David. Thanks for calling, but my finances are a little..."

"Actually, Mom, I'm fine for money. What I need is an answer or two about my fetal development."

"Well, your feet developed well. You had twelve toes, four on each foot, and..."

"No, fetal as in how I was developing while still in the womb. I've just read in the *British Medical Journal* that babies weighing less than 5.5 pounds at birth grow up to be less intelligent than bigger babies, and I couldn't help but wond—"

"Four pounds, seven ounces."

"Umm...?"

"Yes, that would be a smaller number than 5.5, but that doesn't necessarily mean you're stupid. It's just that you were . . . well . . . whenever we played darts, you always asked to play goalie."

"So why was I such a runt? Did you smoke when you were pregnant?"

"Smoked and drank, too, in fact. When we found out I was pregnant we broke out the champagne and celebrated for about six months. We just didn't know any better back then."

"So did you do anything at all to make me a better fetus?"

"Now, dear, you were a fine fetus, better than most. For one thing, you were born in autumn. That meant that you had better nutrition, since I ate more fruits and vegetables during your pregnancy than I would had you been born in the spring. You received a lot more folic acid because of that. Did you know that maternal nutrition during pregnancy may affect the baby's health for life? According to a National Academy of Sciences study, being born in November like you were means that you will actually live longer than if you'd been born in May. If we'd lived in Australia, the reverse is true. You were full of folate as a fetus, and that bodes well for you."

"So I was full of it? Thanks, Mom."

BESIDES AVOIDING alcohol and tobacco, the single best advantage that a fetus can be given is for the mother to have adequate amounts of folic acid in her diet. Half of all birth defects may be a result of folic acid deficiency. The most glaring defect is spina bifida, wherein the spinal cord of the fetus does not close. In addition, heart defects, cleft palates, limb defects, and even urinary tract and stomach anomalies are all less likely to occur in babies whose mothers took adequate amounts of folate. Prenatal folic acid not only reduces the risk of developing childhood cancers, but may also help prevent colorectal cancers when the baby grows up. It is recommended that ALL WOMEN OF CHILD-BEARING AGE TAKE FOLIC ACID SUPPLEMENTATION, particularly since half of all pregnancies are unexpected.

Folic acid comes from foliage in leafy greens the same way that George Bush comes from the bush leagues and brussels sprouts comes from Belgium (where they should remain).

In the late 1990s Canada and the U.S. began fortifying cereal grains, bread, rice, and Domino's pizza with folic acid. Folic acid, being a B vitamin, had to be good for us, right? Some studies even seemed to indicate that large babies who shaved and voted for Dukakis could lower the risk of developing colon and cervical cancer, Alzheimer's disease, and even depression by taking folic acid.

But from the listen-to-what-we-say-but-don't-do-what-we-tell-you files comes the concerning news that too much folic acid may actually screw us up. It has been noted that since the late 1990s there has actually been a rise in colon cancer and that cowboy wannabes in country bars started slapping their own butts while dancing the Macarena. Could folic acid be the culprit? Could supplementing with folic acid help one disease but cause another? Could folic acid cause colon cancer or aggravate it? Could Marie Osmond be wearing dentures?

While many folks take folic acid supplements, I would suggest that, until the colon cancer/folic acid conundrum is resolved, hold off on taking extra folic acid unless you're a woman of child-bearing age.

And to you potential mothers, may the good Lord bless you with a gargantuan baby who will join my dart team.

A LABOUR OF LOVE

"ZOINKER? That's not a word!" I was being Scrabble-challenged and was about to get caught fabricating when I was saved by my yet-to-be-born grandson. My daughter, comfortably leading this stoopid word game, suddenly had an uncomfortable contraction—not the grammatical type, but a contraction of her womb—and the real game was on. She was soon "sentenced" into hard labor, and a baby was about to be born.

As luck would have it, my other daughter, a midwife-in-training who was also calling me a Scrabble cheat, got busy converting our den into a nest! She called in reinforcements and to my surprise, *two* trained midwives showed up at my door with a veritable hospital in tow: oxygen, medications, ivs, week-old tapioca, and more tanks (three) than the Swiss Army.

Four hours later, in one of the sweetest and smoothest births I have ever witnessed, my youngest daughter delivered a nine-pound boy into the hands of my eldest daughter. Not a tear or a tear. A few years ago, I was not a fan of home births, but now, despite my pouting protestations, all of my grandkids have been delivered at home by a midwife. It has been a pleasant revelation to me. Keep in mind I am usually so conservative I consider Pat Buchanan a hippie.

I have always been puzzled why my medical degree, mounted ostentatiously on the wall to prove to my patients, colleagues, and hockey chums that I is an educated doctor, actually declares me a "Doctor of Medicine, Surgery, and Midwifery." Most doctors aren't surgeons, and more would claim having a midriff than being a midwife. When I point this out to others they, too, comment, "I'd never have guessed you had a degree, Dave."

Midwifery has become so popular that a whopping 18 per cent of all births in my city (Victoria, B.C.) are conducted by highly trained midwives. They are experts in delivering great babies, like my entire grand progeny. Based on the principle that low-risk childbirth is a natural process, midwives provide such excellent care and education to mothers that they seldom end up sporting Caesarean scars. They spend a massive amount of time (time most of us midriff types don't have) with the mothers before, during, and after the birth. In my town they perform their art either in a hospital or in the home. Two midwives attend each delivery: one to care for the mother; the other, the baby.

Should a midwife or mother have any concerns at any time in the prenatal care or during labor, they are instantly plugged, so to speak, into an obstetrician, who can work with the midwife at that point.

So now I've become confident discussing the midwifery option with freshly pregnant gals in my office. I have been pleasantly surprised by how many return months later to thank me for directing them to a great pregnancy and birth experience.

So let's give these midwives their due date. They certainly deliver.

With my daughters busy delivering, I returned to the Scrabble table alone and made a few surreptitious changes to win the game, a victory I have dedicated to my new grandson—Zoinker.

NAVEL ACADEMICS

On rare occasions, doctors get into trouble with the medical authorities as a result of complaints from patients. For me this occurs on Tuesdays. A nostalgic tear wells up in my eye as I recall, oh so well, the first time I was hauled up on the carpet. I was a brash young intern ("intern" meaning that we are interned and entombed within a hospital—we are not yet able to set up practice and get sued for real).

"So, young intern, who we presume would ultimately like to make a living as a doctor, would you care to explain why you said what you did?"

It had been a dark and stormy night, and I had been on maternity call roughly 478 hours. I was minutes away from catching another baby in the labor and delivery room, this time courtesy of a woman from Gabriola Island.

Gabriola is a gorgeous little pearl in the Gulf Island necklace that adorns the waters between Vancouver Island and the B.C. mainland. It is home to many a free spirit, including many Americans who spirited themselves free of the draft. It remains the happy hippie home of gumboots, granola, and good guano. It is the land of tie-dye, bandanas, vw vans, and peace. The birth of this freshest Gabriolan was going well, though a naked four-year-old prancing about the room sticking his nose into the action site (to check for his new sib) was a tad distracting.

Fifteen minutes after Moonshadow Raccoon Nosehair pleasantly entered the world came the placenta (afterbirth).

"Could you save that for us please, doctor?"

"Why?" I inquired.

"Well, we plan to cook it up and eat it," they replied.

Honestly believing that they were kidding, I then let loose with a wisecrack that subsequently landed me in hot water. "So, what do you cook it with, Placenta Helper?"

Such was my first exposure to placentaphagia (the eating of placenta). According to the Julia Childproducts cookbook *Quick and Easy Human Organs*, the placenta can be fried, sautéed, fricasseed, and even baked (half-baked?). The February 1999 edition of *Harper's Magazine* actually describes some popular recipes for placenta. Honest.

Various cultures are known to spread the placenta in gardens. Others bury it with a palm seedling, which, upon maturing as a tree, can be a reminder to the child that part of them is in part of that coconut.

In addition to being used as a dietary delicacy, protein- and hormone-rich placenta is used in health care products ranging from shampoos to Chinese remedies for impotence, menopause, and general anti-aging. Those with an extra $25,000 (i.e., those who don't buy the same stocks I do) who wish to feel younger may wish to undergo placental injections.

Placenta, which is derived from the same stem cells as the baby, is the only non-diseased live organ that can be removed from the body for study. Most folks outside of West Virginia resent having a liver or brain removed for scientific study. Placentologists are able to use this organ to test drugs or poisons, extract hormones, investigate disease (genetic), and even use the placental membrane for healing burn wounds.

It is remarkable to realize that, be it an inny or an outie, the wee lint collector in the middle of our belly was once our life-line. We can be born sans various appendages and even organs, but everyone (with the exception of Adam and Eve, perhaps?) has a navel base. The placenta does not actually transmit mother's blood to baby, but rather it acts as a barrier preventing her blood from mixing with that of the fetus. It selectively allows the passage of substances required for fetal development, including nutrients, oxygen, and Snickers bars. It is also the conduit for returning waste products like ammonia and broccoli to the mother. If this eighteen-ounce organ gets infected, has a diminished blood supply, is contaminated by alcohol or tobacco, or is not sitting in its proper locale within the womb, then the fetus is at risk of having birth defects.

By examining the placenta, known as the "diary of life," much about life in the womb can be determined. Cerebral palsy (brain damage caused by a "botched" birth) is a major reason that 80 per cent of obstetricians have been sued. Much to the chagrin of lawyers, there may not necessarily be anyone to blame in many of these cases. The placenta, rather than the doctor, may be the culprit, or it may reveal an answer as to the real cause of brain damage. My own obvious brain damage is likely due to the fact that I was born . . . on a Tuesday.

CALLING YOUR SHOTS

I recall sitting with my mother in a veterinarian's office with our Rottweiler-Doberman-Mike Tyson cross, Petunia. I was busy studying the latest *Spider-Man* comic while Petunia was trying to gnaw through his Hannibal Lecter muzzle in order to better scratch 'n' sniff or maul 'n' ingest the skittish waiting room clients. Suddenly, around the corner wheeled the nurse of my dreams.

"Hi, my name's Kitty. What's his?"

"Petunia," my mother replied. "Pet for short."

"No, I mean your son."

"Oh, David. He's going to be a doctor one day."

"Really, how old is he?"

"Thirty-seven."

"No, the dog."

"Oh, three."

"Is he fixed?"

"Who?" replied my mother, a concerned furrow puckering her brow.

"I see he slobbers quite a bit. Does he do any tricks?"

"Well, he knows a little magic . . ."

"No, I mean the dog."

By the time the interview was over, I was so confused I wasn't sure if I was free of fleas, house-trained, or liked my belly rubbed. But we were really stumped by the question, "Has he had all his shots?" I'm not certain how the confusion was finally sorted out, but I do know that to this day I have never had heartworms or distemper (though I once threw a tantrum when *Josie and the Pussycats* was canceled). Petunia has never had the mumps or whooping cough.

Confusion still reigns in the world of vaccinations.

Have you had all your shots? Are you even aware of what they are now? Should you have more? Should you have less? Are you up to date on all your shots?

As more new and exciting vaccines are added to the regimen of a child's life (now thirty-seven vaccinations for eleven diseases), doctors are facing hard questions from parents—questions like: "Why should we expose little Orenthal here to the risk of vaccination side effects when chicken pox is such a mild disease?" and "What is the capital of Uzbekistan?"

Vaccination has become a victim of its own success. There are those who mistakenly feel that diseases such as polio or diphtheria appear to be eradicated, hence vaccination is no longer necessary. Why must we start filling our kids up with vaccines as soon as they are hatched? But in 1990, after an easing-up in measles vaccinations, the usual 1,500 cases of measles per year in the U.S. ballooned to 55,000 cases. Hundreds were hospitalized, and 132 unvaccinated children died. In addition, every pediatrician, it seems, can recall a horror story involving an unvaccinated infant who contracted pertussis.

And so, yes, vaccination remains a cornerstone of public health.

So let's review why it's important to remain vigilant in developing herd immunity (meaning all us cows must be vaccinated to prevent the bug from getting in among us) in the battle against disease. Several vaccines are now routinely offered in childhood. They include:

- *Diphtheria:* With only five cases a year in North America, vaccination has all but wiped out this dreaded and dangerous disease.
- *Polio:* A once-devastating paralyzing illness that claimed FDR among its victims, polio is now very close to becoming the next disease that will join smallpox on the eradicated list. Though there have been no wild cases in North America since 1979, a few pockets, such as a recent outbreak in Haiti, still exist. The amazing polio story of Salk and Sabin has resulted in virtual vaccination victory over a very vicious virus.
- *Pertussis:* Under fire for years, the controversial "whooping cough" vaccine has been associated with the most significant side effects. However, a recent changeover to the new acellular vaccine has made pertussis vaccination safe. Nasty outbreaks of pertussis still occur. Whooping cough can be tricky to detect. It doesn't always have a WHOOP, THERE IT IS presentation, and so this disease can be easily missed and readily spread. Doctors often refer to it as the "whoopsing cough"—as in "Whoops, sorry, I thought it was just a cold." Pertussis in an adult can be an annoying, persistent cough, but to an infant it can be life-threatening. It's still under discussion whether or not adults should be re-immunized in order to avoid becoming pertussis reservoirs.

- *HiB:* Haemophilus influenzea type b vaccine is another marvelous vaccination success story. It was introduced in the 1990s as a routine immunization. Where HiB meningitis killed 5 per cent and left another 25 per cent of its 12,000 annual victims brain-damaged, the HiB vaccine is already close to making this common form of childhood meningitis a disease of the past.
- *Meningococcal:* Protects against a meningitis so dangerous that, when not fatal, it often leads to brain damage.
- *Hepatitis B:* Hep B as in HepBurn does indeed burn the liver and is the leading cause of liver cancer. The first vaccine (of what will hopefully be many) that protects against cancer.
- *Tetanus:* Though there are now only fifty to one hundred cases of "lockjaw" per year in North America, 30 per cent of those who contract tetanus will die. A booster (along with diphtheria) every ten years is recommended for everyone but Petunia. Lockjaw would certainly save on muzzles.
- *Measles:* A once common, now rare disease in the well-vaccinated Americas, measles still kills more than 1.5 million children annually worldwide. Encephalitis (infection of the brain) leading to brain damage is a complication of measles, mumps, and even chicken pox. This ten-cent vaccine could save billions of dollars and millions of lives, were it a priority globally.
- *Mumps:* More dangerous than measles, mumps can cause an even higher rate of encephalitis (brain damage) and death than measles. Immunization has dropped the number of cases in the U.S. from 200,000 in 1968 to 906 in 1995. Outbreaks do still occur, usually initiated by the unvaccinated. A rave party, for example, caused an outbreak in Vancouver, B.C., in 1997.

   "Hey, dude, pick your brain damage: Ecstasy, crystal meth, or mumps?"

   "Kewl!"
- *Rubella:* Also known as German measles, this viral infection is basically measles with an accent. Vaccination is meant to decrease this disease in order to protect the fetuses in the herd

from some very destructive defects. All pregnant women are screened to ensure that they already have antibodies to rubella. Complications include numerous horrible defects, including blindness, heart malformations, and an overwhelming desire to inhale copious amounts of wiener schnitzel while dancing the polka.

- *Chicken pox:* Chicken pox? Yes. Now part of routine childhood immunization programs in the U.S., the varicella vaccine is given along with the MMR (measles, mumps, and rubella) at age twelve months. A simple blood test can detect whether or not you are immune to varicella. If not, strongly consider becoming so. Some of the sickest, most uncomfortable people I have seen are adults with chicken pox. With their bodies and brains covered in painful sores, varicella victims are a miserable lot. This very safe vaccine can prevent the potentially fatal complications of this pox, including encephalitis, pneumonia, growth of tail feathers, and even necrotizing fasciitis ("flesh-eating disease"). Chicken pox kills about one hundred people a year in North America and hospitalizes another ten thousand. Still, some in our herd are too chicken to get the shot.

- *Pneumococcus:* Given at two, four, six, and twelve months, this vaccine prevents pneumonias, meningitis, ear infections, conjunctivitis (pinkeye), and sinusitis caused by the group of bacteria known as pneumococcus. There are more than ninety serotypes of pneumococcus; all adults over age sixty-five are given a shot that covers twenty-three of the worst types. Children now get a shot that covers the seven deadliest childhood pneumococci. In addition, with increasing concerns of mutant antibiotic-resistant bugs, this vaccine will actually work to decrease drug resistance. With more children immunized, bacteria will be carried by fewer people. Antibiotic usage will drop off, and bacteria will have less opportunity to develop resistance.

What a bright herd we are.

PLUMP PUFFY PROGENY

Should doctors be healthy role models for our youth? If we aren't, should we lose our jobs? Recently a raft of rather rotund doctors in Austria's state-run clinics with a BMI (body mass index) over twenty-five received letters telling them to shape up, or they'd be fired. Fired for being fat. Fired for being a roll model.

One in three kids in North America is overweight, while a Big Whoppering 9 million kids are classified as obese. Pediatric obesity is the greatest health threat facing our children. Some, unfortunately, are primed to be large, as a genetic battle between hormones like ghrelin and leptin is waged in the internal milieu. But many others, the corpulent computer-keystered Krispy Kremed kids, are also developing a host of co-morbid conditions associated with obesity that, up until now, have never been heard of in children. A life sentence of misery resulting from Type II diabetes is showing up in younger and younger kids. More recently NASH (non-alcoholic steato hepatitis), previously a purview of plump, portly, or puffy parents, is now showing up in obese youth and damaging their livers. Twelve-year-old livers are looking like they've been abused in the navy (motto: "We Sail Wet") for twenty years.

A few tips on how to prevent your young 'un from becoming a big 'un:

1. The best thing for an obese child: give him a prescription for a new set of parents. Studies indicate that many parents with obese kids, especially overweight boys, see their child through rose-colored glasses and don't see the "big" problem. "Porky's not obese, doctor, he's just big-boned. Now you've upset him. There, there, now, you're mommy's little piglet. Have another Oreo, and don't listen to that Austrian."

2. "Remember that breast is best." Another navy motto, but also refers to the fact that the GUTS (Growing Up Today Study) found that children who had been breastfed were 34 per cent less likely

to become obese, regardless of how chubby or diabetic their mother is. Of course, if your big baby is twenty-seven years old, then perhaps he's just best left fat.

3. Know the difference between role model and roll model. "Okay kid, go out and do some push-ups or something, just leave me alone, and keep away from my remote!" Kids born to overweight moms are fifteen times more likely to be obese by age six, and in fact start to pack on the Gerbers by age three.

4. Remove words like "fat," "exercise," and "diet," and replace them with more fun euphemisms like "play," "great nutrition," and "kumquat." (Kumquat has nothing to do with this topic; I just think it's a hilarious word.)

5. Don't eat in front of the TV; in fact, get rid of your TV. Go ahead. In fact, if you have a fifty-two-inch LCD then, as a caring medical professional, I think it would be in your best interest for me to remove that from your home. Trust me. I am thinking only of you, your children, and the play-offs.

6. Eat as a family.

7. Eat like the French: slow, all-day lunches with excessive amounts of wine. I believe this works because the diners pass out and don't wake up in time to eat supper. Make the meal a marathon, not a sprint. Try to stretch out the meal, or you'll stretch out your Lululemons.

8. Start meals with salad or soup. Stuff 'em early, stuff 'em hard! (They won't be able to wolf down dessert.)

9. Keep your fridge full of healthy snacks like carrot sticks, celery sticks, and Snickers sticks. Obesity comes not only from eating the wrong things, but from not eating the right things. Undernourished kids gain weight as they get hungry and end up eating cardboard-like products.

10. Don't keep junk food in the house. Changing eating habits as a child is easier than treating obesity as an adult. I might add that nowhere on the Snickers wrapper does it actually refer to itself as a junk food, per se.

11. Be active in promoting active lifestyle options for kids in your community.
12. Let kids get their sleep. Leptin, a good-guy hormone, is released during sleep.
13. Move to Vienna.

IN-YOUR-EYE-SIS

Ever had "The Dream"? You know, the one where the Swedish flight attendan... er... the one when you're standing in a forest and you have to piddle so desperately that your molars are doing the backstroke, and the little red alarm in your bladder is screaming "flood warning?" And so, to great relief, you put out the fire, emptying the kidney's pride and joy into the forest flora. Relief is replaced by grief when you wake to find that "the dream" is now "the pool."

What if waking to a soaking wet bed was a nightly occurrence? To millions of kids and even thousands of adults, it is.

Nocturnal enuresis (pronounced "in-your-eye-sis") refers to nighttime urinary incontinence.

Fifteen per cent of five-year-olds, 7 per cent of seven-year-olds and 1 to 2 per cent of teenagers suffer from the emotionally (and bladder-) draining problem of bedwetting.

True or false?

1. Bedwetting is a psychological problem associated with abnormally deep sleep.
   False. This has not been shown to be the case, although most of these kids are deep sleepers. Counseling does little, if any, good for the actual problem, but can help deal with the emotional aftermath. One camp counselor in Oregon used to gather the bedwetters together at night and after a pep talk would actually have the kids stand up and say, "My name is Joe, and I wet the bed."

2. Restricting fluid helps.
   False. Makes little difference.
3. If both parents had bedwetting problems, there is a 78 per cent chance their kids will. If one parent had a problem, a 44 per cent chance.
   True. It appears that unlucky chromosome 13 is the genetic link that allows bedwetting to "run" in families. A sort of missing leak link.
4. Hormones are a culprit.
   True. Tonight, as you enter the world of the dreamweaver, a little hormone called vasopressin will be set loose in your system. It will tell your kidneys to call it a day and quit making all that urine. Many kids have yet to develop the necessary amount of vasopressin, and so, in the middle of the night, they spring a leak.
5. Drugs should be used to stop bedwetting.
   True. Though drugs do not cure the problem, a little vasopressin nasal spray, called DDAVP (also available in pill form) usually stops bedwetting dead in its tracks. This is highly useful at important times like that sleepover, going to camp, or bedding down at Grandma's.

The most successful technique in dealing with enuresis remains the bell-and-pad early missile warning system. This alarming device is clipped onto the underwear near the source of the Nile. DO NOT hook it onto any portion of the anatomy. The general idea is that as soon as Junior begins to release that first drop, the moisture will trigger a loud alarm. Junior will instantly stop, and Mother will peacefully enter the room and escort Junior to the commode, where the appreciative young fellow will thank his mother, empty his bladder, and return to bed and back to the dream of standing in a forest with nothing to do.

But the reality of the situation is that when this harsh Stephen King–designed alarm screeches (soon to be released on the next

Mötley Crüe album), Junior is so terrorized that his testicles usually withdraw to the general vicinity of his tonsils. The parents bolt out of bed and, while Dad clings to the ceiling by his fingernails, Mom is running about with the fire extinguisher spraying in all directions. Junior is finally located rocking back and forth in the fetal position, tearing at the Chinese New Year fireworks going off in his crotch.

When assisting in surgery, I will often turn my pager to "vibrate" mode to help keep the OR quiet and not wake the anesthetist. Usually, the pager sits on my belt, often right over a nerve in my groin. When it goes off, the electric jolt in my nether regions causes me to pitch forward, scalpel swinging wildly. Now a similar new vibrating alarm exists for Junior, called the Potty Pager. It sends a vibrating warning to him when he starts to wet. Junior trundles off to fix the leak, parents sleep, and Grandma rolls over.

WORMOLOGY

Took my son on a fishing expedition recently. Wanted to teach him the finer points of how trout avoid the bait of even the best fishermen. Before heading off into the wilds, we stopped at a fine dining establishment for a final meal of non-fish, him secure in the knowledge that we would catch the rest of our meals, me secure in the knowledge that I was about to shed a few pounds. While waiting for our meal, he zipped across the street to a sports store to pick up some bait. Bursting back into the restaurant, he called out, "Dad, I've got worms!" Funny how quiet Burger King can become while diners rearrange their seating.

But many of you reading this book also have worms and just don't know it. In fact, one billion (that is a "B" as in Bummer) of you faithful readers are host to a large roundworm called Ascaris. (See below. . . um, in the chapter.) And while you think this only refers to readers in Beijing and Calcutta, let me remind you that

45 million North Americans share their daily dietary dinners and Ding Dongs with pinworms.

Pinworms
These wee white wigglers infest 10 per cent of all kids and, while not harmful in any way, they can create an annoying anal itch that can lead to some less-than-socially-acceptable (unless you're out fishing with your dad) attempts to rect-ify the itch. At night, the female pinworm leaves her happy colonic home, pops out the anus, airs out her laundry, takes a few fresh breaths, and lays a few eggs. (I get royalties if this idea gets picked up by Disney.) This creates the annoying nocturnal itch that causes Junior to fidget while trying to fall asleep. This also proves my point that it is not always the male who is a pain in that part of the nether regions.

To definitively prove the presence of pinworms, wait until the patient/victim falls asleep. Equip yourself with a flashlight, Scotch tape, and Marlin Perkins. If you shine your light and catch the female worm wide-eyed in your beam, then you've made the diagnosis. Do not shoot; this is an illegal hunting method. While this may not be the most dignified thing you've ever done, how many of you have actually watched *Jerry Springer?*

If you see no worm or anything else that ruins your evening, then place the tape on the anal area, thus removing the microscopic eggs. This, again, is best done while Junior sleeps; otherwise, he is quite apt to run screaming to the neighbors each time you reach for the Scotch tape. He could very well go catatonic when his schoolteacher takes Scotch tape out of her desk. Place the tape on a slide and then take the tape to your doctor (after lunch, please).

To avoid pinworm eggs, scrub your hands and fingernails (eggs love to get in here) before eating, discourage nail biting and thumb sucking, and keep fingernails short. My own mother used to clip my nails so short that my cuticles disappeared, but we saved on Scotch tape.

Tapeworms
Speaking of tape, these flatworms whose larvae we might ingest from inadequately cooked beef, pork, or fish can live quietly for years deep within the bowels of our... well... bowels. A heavy worm load, however, may cause a slow anemia or be the cause of chronic diarrhea.

Ascaris
While living in the South Pacific, I got to know these slimy monsters quite well. The largest of the roundworms, these worms can grow up to twelve inches in length. Their life cycle is straight out of a Hitchcock horror film, *Psycho Worms*. The human host swallows an egg. Larvae hatch in the bowel and then penetrate the bowel wall and head for the lungs. From there, they climb up the windpipe and are swallowed by the host, where they descend merrily into the small intestine. There they mature and lay up to 200,000 eggs per day. Not only did I frequently see patients vomit revolting masses of these worms, but I also found them stuck in a patient's appendix, causing appendicitis.

"Dad, how come those trout didn't bite?" lamented my son after our trip.

"Sorry, son, but we fished perfectly, you just had a bad case of worms."

NIT WIT
Head lice. (I suspect that 42 per cent of you have already begun scratching.)

Though a louse is barely the size of a pinhead, medical school professors delight in illustrating the 60,000,000x magnified photo of the beast, a frightful behemoth that best resembles an extra from the set of *Jurassic Park*. Half the class wakes up and starts scratching wildly, while the rest make a dash for the exits.

The louse, which needs to feed on your blood to survive, enjoys several snacks a day. The saliva that it injects into your skin through its sucking jaws prevents the blood from clotting. It is the saliva that causes that infamous itch. The timorous wee lousie lays an average of five eggs (called "nits" by their mothers) per day. Needing warmth, the nits are laid at the very base of the hair root, where they are then glued onto the hair using a combination of Krazy Glue, Velcro, and Portland cement.

(By now I suspect 78 per cent of you are spraying your scalps with industrial-strength Raid.)

A female louse lives only about a month. During that time it goes through puberty, meets a male louse (redundant?), falls mitely in love, gets hitched, pays exorbitant taxes to other blood-sucking groups, raises a family on Hilton Head, and has about 150 lousey kids (your basic nits), all while using your scalp as both home and food supply.

Nits, the white, oval, waxy egg sacs, take about a week to hatch. The louse usually inhabits the nape of the neck, a spot behind the ears, or the White House. It cannot fly, nor can it jump, swim, or drive (no lice-ense). Head-to-head collision is the favored mode of transport.

So do the math. One female louse, 150 offspring, all ready to lay their own 150 nits. In no time you have an entire jungle teeming with Jurassic lice and nits! Small children are hiding in the scalp kitchens! Raptors and *T. rex* are battling to the death just above your ears!... you get the idea. Basically, you're an egg-head. (By now I suspect that 96 per cent of you have immersed your heads in a vat of boiling oil.)

A dirty disease, you say? Oddly enough, lice have been found to prefer clean, fine hair rather than dandruffy or dirty hair, as I tried to explain in vain to my mother before she scrubbed the scalp right off my head. They also have an odd preference for red-heads and brunettes. They could care less about blondes. (Fools.)

Treatment

1. Kill the lice and nits. Remember that most of the commercial preparations are toxic pesticides and not Vidal Sassoon hair care

products. Be careful. Do *not* use them when you get an itchy scalp or mistake a flake of dandruff for a nit. Most of the preparations will kill both lice and nits older than four days old. Fresh nits younger than four days have no nervous system and will not succumb until they get one. Thus, a second treatment seven days later will usually nail those raptors. Malathion products are more successful than some of the other pest killers. Use leftovers for dandelions or tax collectors.

2. Speaking of eternal pests, the nits must be completely removed, tedious as it is. Get close to the roots with a very fine comb. Comb often and comb early, and go after the ones closest to the scalp. The nits farther away are hatched already. Add conditioner or olive oil to make it easier. Use leftover combs to play juice harp.

3. Speaking of olive oil, applying this clogs up lice lungs and finishes off the lice that the pesticide doesn't get. Use leftover oil for cooking or head immersion.

4. Speaking of cooking, an intriguing device called a LouseBuster cooks and dries out the lice like a fancy hair dryer. Use leftover dried lice for show and tell.

5. Speaking of drying, a louse dries up and dies after no more than twenty hours off a human scalp. Vacuum hard, and fire all linens and clothing into hot water. What can't be washed (stuffed toys, boys of the male gender) needs to be bagged up and set aside for a couple of weeks. Use resistant leftover boys for chores.

6. Speaking of resistance, a well-founded concern has risen concerning resistance to pesticide shampoos, giving birth to "super lice." This worry has also launched several home remedies and "suffocants," including mayonnaise and Vaseline. My advice is to hold the mayo (my mother always made me put the mayo in the fridge, warning that I could die of warm mayo disease unless I was treated at the Mayo Clinic). Vaseline is even harder to get out of your hair than the nits. If the lice seem refractory to treatment, keep at it with the combs, try a different pesticide, or amputate your hair. (By now, all of you are scrubbing your scalps with steel wool while firing up the acetylene blowtorch.)

WHERE'S WALDO'S LOCKJAW

I am not a well-read man, unless you include literary classics like *Archie and Jughead Get Haircuts in Kentucky* or *The Exciting History of Maple Syrup.* So my recent venture into the town of Concord, Massachusetts, to visit the famed battle site of the American Revolution, turned out to be a blistering shock to my ego. While every tourist in town was excited about the Shot Heard Round the World, it appeared they were equally thrilled by the fact that Ralph Waldo Emerson, Henry David Thoreau, Louisa May Alcott, and Nathaniel (Mother forgot a middle name) Hawthorne all hailed from this one small New England town. I, too, was caught up in the excitement of visiting their homes/museums, paying homage to their nail clippings, etc. until I realized that I had actually never read any of their books. While I have been known on occasion to Belittle Women, and I can usually find Waldo in my son's college picture books, I have never knowingly turned a page written by these literary giants. So I decided to correct this obvious defect in my culture and at least go swimming in the apparently famous Walden Pond.

The plaque beside the replica cabin of Henry Thoreau learned me that Thoreau was so devastated by his brother's death from tetanus that he decided he would isolate himself from the civilized world and go and live in Winnipeg, er... Walden for two years and write great books. Tetanus! At last, something in Concord I had read about.

The next time you head to the doctor to fix up that gouge you sustained while playing a game of William Tell with One-Eyed Carl, you will be asked when your last tetanus shot was. You will either reply, "I don't remember" if you are honest or "last week" if the sight of a needle makes your SpongeBob boxers quiver. The doctor will then administer a wee booster shot that will cover you against tetanus for ten years.

But why? Is tetanus a common or horrible disease? Does anybody die of tetanus? Certainly none of my patients have; at least, they have never admitted it. But tetanus, a.k.a. lockjaw, used to be feared and dreaded, killing more than 90 per cent of those who contracted it. In 1947 universal tetanus immunization along with a booster each decade was introduced in North America, and lockjaw has all but become a problem of the past. Now fewer than fifty cases a year occur in North America, with about 10 per cent of those succumbing to the disease.

Be aware that growing in the soil right next to YOUR HOUSE are little evil bacteria known as *Clostridium tetani*. Get one of those guys into a cut and, should you not be immunized, you may soon develop a painful spasm in your jaw and neck. This spasm, known as trismus, stiffens the face, giving it the look of Jack Nicholson in his role as the Joker or Joan Rivers in her role as Joan Rivers. Lockjaw can progress swiftly, turning into lock-body as the spasm travels to all your muscles, rendering you as stiff as my son's hair on Saturday night. Soil with a high manure content, found at farms and government grounds, is loaded with these tetanus spores, which pass safely through cattle.

But more than 500,000 deaths occur worldwide from tetanus each year, many of them newborn babes who contract tetanus from having their umbilical cord cut under non-sterile conditions. Hardly a great start to life, and one that underscores our need to lend our expertise, wealth, and compassion to suffering fifth-world countries. In North America, the five or six tetanus deaths a year occur in those who have not been immunized or had a booster. While this represents a death rate of about 10 per cent, it is a far cry from the 91 per cent death rate that those who contracted lockjaw in Thoreau's time sustained. So make certain you're not that one Waldo in a million, and go get boosterized.

SKATERDUDES

Skateboarding is PAIN personified. A skateboarding park recently opened up around the corner from my clinic. This has added color (primarily red) to my practice and hipness to my vocabulary. With no shortage of fractured this and lacerated that now skating through my office door, I have become, unofficially, the doctor to these cement-surfin' sons of stitches.

"Yo, doctor dude, I was carvin' some phat air, like I was totally amped, bro, when I ate it and bought me this gnarlacious swellbow."

Translated: "My elbow hurts."

What has surprised me is that these swellbow, tweaker, and hipper victims are not only sixteen-year-old baggy-pant boarders, but also dudes and dudettes in their twenties and thirties who actually hold jobs that don't require supersizing stuff. In fact, 170 of the injured North American skateboarders hospitalized last year were over age sixty-five!

And so, I have decided to give the wheels a go. Sort of. My sons, with a twinkle in their eyes, convinced me that I should try rollerblading, a sport that I have eschewed, possibly due to the frequency with which rollerbladers end up on the hood of my car with relatively little effort on my behalf. And for a life-long hockey player, inline skates are frightening. Stopping on ice skates means a quick turn to the side. Doing the same thing on rollers means a quick trip to the hospital. And so it was that with six hundred pounds of armor draped about my joints, head, and any skin that I might possibly protect from the local asphalt, I teetered on these blades like a newborn giraffe on ice. "Cow-abunga, Dad!" My fear of these wheels of death was validated when I met my first speed bump at ramming speed. Unable to brake, I was promptly launched horizontally headlong, landing with an unceremonious splat and coming to a halt only after deploying my elbows as brakes. First day, first swellbow, a condition known to the uncool as bursitis of the elbow.

At least I didn't have a hipper or a tweaker. More than 100,000 injured skateboarders show up in the emergency room, a third of whom have less than one week's experience. Most experienced boarders treat themselves, usually by punching their heads repeatedly until the injury hurts less than their head. Skaters suffer some significant smacks to the skull, followed by broken wrists, faces, and ankles. Treating these brazen but broken boardin' boppers requires first learning their lingo.

Hipper: "Yo, doctor dude, I got this outrageous hipper from goofy-footin' into a fakie."

To inspect a patient's hip, some clothing must be removed, but given the skaters' sartorial tastes, this is rarely required.

"Yep, I can see it from here, you have a traumatic greater trochanteric bursitis."

"Whoa, awesome! Can I keep skating, or do I play Sega for a while?"

Reach down to where you think your hip is located. Feel that bony thing jutting out? (If not, consider Atkins.) This is the infamous greater trochanter, a part of the femur covered in a fluid-filled sac called a bursa, which acts as a shock absorber to prevent muscle from rubbing up against bone. Bump this too hard or lie on it too long and the bursa will be traumatized and will swell and hurt. If it doesn't get better on its own, then a well-placed cortisone shot works wonders.

Swellbow: Another bodacious bursa sits over the bony part of the bent elbow. The olecranon bursa is easily traumatized, as well as easily infected. This swollen bursa (bursitis) blows up like a blowfish and feels like a jug of water has been taped to the victim's arm. I will often drain these and place a pressure dressing on them (or they fill right back up). If they do fill back up, a cortisone injection may keep infection at bay. An infected bursa, however, is a serious bummer given its proximity to the joint.

Tweaker: Kickflip down a rail or fall on an outstretched hand and you may suffer several serious injuries to the wrist. You may fracture one of eight wrist bones, the scaphoid bone being the most dangerous. The fracture may not be obvious, but persistent pain where the thumb joins the wrist (the snuffbox) is highly suspicious. More than a wrist tweaker, if a fractured scaphoid is not set properly, you may be in for some real gnarly surgery.

Yep, these skaters have brought some outrageous injuries into my clinic, and for that . . . I am totally stoked.

THE UPSIDE OF DOWN'S

I suspected the patient I was to see was female, given that I was making rounds on the female ward of my jungle hospital on the island of Tanna in the remote South Pacific. It was not always easy to determine which occupant of the bed was intended for my Western cures. As was wont to occur, three people of assorted gender were sprawled on the bed and two more, including the patient, were sleeping on a grass mat underneath it. All were family members of Elisabeth, a twelve-year-old burn victim, who had been dancing around the fire in her grass skirt. The skirt ignited, and Elisabeth had burns to more than 35 per cent of her young body. The Tannese had a silly habit of staying with family members who were ill until they either died or "came good again." With no place to stay at the hospital but on or under the bed (a novelty item in Tanna) or outside under a tree, the family was hunkered down for the two months Elisabeth was with us.

Elisabeth had Down syndrome. I was astonished to see that, simply because she had an extra chromosome, she was in some way extra important to the Tannese. Far from being embarrassed by her syndrome, they relished the opportunity to be with her, and adored her as though she were a prized mango. The highlight of my daily rounds was checking on a perpetually smiling Elisabeth and her doting family. Patiently, they nursed this happy cherub back to health, carrying her down a treacherous hillside twice a day to soak in their Lourdes, the salt water of the Coral Sea.

I was often struck by the differences between our "civilized" society and the "primitive" Tannese people of Vanuatu. The Ni-Vanuatu people would be shocked to know that civilized society often screen fetuses to ensure that any fetus with Down syndrome will never see the light of day.

Every parent hopes for a baby with ten fingers, ten toes, and forty-six chromosomes, twenty-three each from the mother and the maleman. Sadly, having an extra chromosome 21 (as occurs every thousand conceptions) means the child will have DS and, in some cases, be considered undesirable. As we bend over backward to be politically tolerant of anyone with a loud lobby group, we usually condemn those with DS as faulty and often terminate their lives before they even get started. Undoubtedly, raising a DS child is difficult. It consumes more time, demands more patience, and tests character. To those of you who lovingly meet the daily challenges of raising any disabled child, I say to you, you are heroes. You are *my* heroes. One kindhearted couple I'm aware of has adopted eight unwanted DS children.

In addition to being mentally challenged and sporting a facial look that labels them as different or deficient, the DS child will often have significant hearing difficulties and severe heart problems. But are they defective humans?

There is an upside to Down's. A huge upside.

They smile too much.

They are openly affectionate.

They are forgiving to the point that even after being mercilessly taunted, they will turn and say, "He is my best friend."

They are trustworthy and trusting.

They are happy, honest, and guileless.

They are kindness, goodness, and benevolence personified.

They are not a mistake. They are a gift.

They are different, not defective, and as one mother noted, "as a violet in a field of daisies is different. They are still beautiful flowers. We should not be trying to make them into daisies, but rather we should cherish these violets for what they are." In fact, we can all enrich our own lives by looking for opportunities to serve those who live and work with DS. We can provide respite and patronize businesses that hire those with DS. We can smile back. We can welcome the enchantment of chromosome 21.

BACK AWAY

(*from the* TONGUE)

DEPRESSORS

THANKS FOR THE BILL

I could always tell when Bill was in the waiting room. His telltale bullhorn honk and blow preceded a loud, guttural reach into the bottom of his lungs that would expectorate that last piece of inhaled microbial mass. This would usually garner stares of revulsion and comments of utter disgust, primarily from his wife. Bill had a few ongoing medical problems. In addition to a chronic cough, he battled depression, but one would never have known, given his upbeat, jovial demeanor and back-slapping as he entered the exam room. I would slap his back in return, partly hoping to dislodge the alien that appeared to be jammed somewhere deep in the roots of his bronchial tree.

His appointment was always punctuated with "Doc, you're the greatest" a couple of times each visit. Before he left there was a quick *yet manly* "How about a hug, doc, you're the greatest." Bill was good for the ego and soothing to the soul.

Bill was poor. Dirt poor. Can't-buy-new-socks poor. Formerly he was a galley slave, a navy cook who now couldn't get work doing what he loved but rather ended up cleaning kitchens all night long so that the working cooks could come in and prepare food in ways that Bill never approved of. He was a little bitter about that. His three teenage sons were a concern to him, as he didn't want them to feel poor. But every second visit, Bill would bring me a gift. A ball cap he had found on a bus, a coupon from one of the restaurants he cleaned, a belt or a tie. He had no money. I have always recalled the words of an accountant who commented that he had clients who made small fortunes yet contributed little if anything to charity. Little money or little thought..These types of people hoard their gains and will clutch on to them until they die, if not longer.

Bill's cough turned into lung cancer, years of smoking in the galleys of the navy ships, ashes spilling from his cigarette into the soup of the day, cream of Marlboro. The day I revealed this to him, I was met with the expected flood of tears from his wife. Bill, initially stunned, recovered quickly with, "I knew you'd find out what was wrong with me. You're the best, doc."

Yeah, sure, Bill, I did a great job.

"Doc, how long do I have?"

Not long.

The next week he returned with his Disneyland-bound sisters, who decided they would take him to his heaven on Earth before he was taken to his heaven off Earth.

"I've always wanted to go to Disneyland, doc. Can I go?"

Sure, Bill, but don't delay.

"I won't take any really long rides, doc. How about a hug?"

The cancer did the usual lung cancer thing and spread voraciously. It was killing Bill too quickly. There is no miracle cure for lung cancer. Bill died. People wept. I am a people. I thought of how poor impoverished Bill now has the same amount of money in his pocket as the kazillionaire who inevitably dies: bupkis.

Back at the office, there was a gift waiting for me. It was from Bill—a beautiful, expensive mahogany-framed picture. This gorgeous Disneyland memento adorns my wall today. It is a pencil sketch of one of the seven dwarfs. You guessed it . . . Doc.

START YOUR ENGINES

My car, worth about $86.43 when the tank is full, recently required really radical surgery followed by a couple of days in the expensive scare unit. During my bayside vigil I noticed that most of the other sick cars were older models, and it dawned on me that cars are much like patients, just as medics are a lot like mechanics. Doctors mimic mechanics by wearing outfits with their names embroidered proudly over their hearts, hanging interesting anatomy pictures on their walls (usually without the stiletto heels), and, in attempting to diagnose assorted rattles, performing several unnecessary and expensive tests. But sick patients mimic cars, a sort of auto-immune thing.

CARS	PATIENTS
sedans	sedentary
fan belts may stretch	Dairy Queen meets Burger King
needs more grease	supersize them fries, will ya?
may require expensive bodywork	the future is plastics
battery tests	battery of tests
if no regulator, then must use crank	cranky if not regular

seats may sag when vehicle is old and worn

lights don't always come on,

no matter how you try and flip the switch

looks better when waxed

more sluggish in winter

can cram a lot of groceries into some larger vehicles

defective computer	fuzzy computer
and fuzzy dice	and gambling addiction
smoking may indicate	smoking may indicate

CARS	PATIENTS
brake fluid leak	brain fluid leak
fueled with high octane gas	Taco Time
comes to screeching halt when overheated	menopause
leather upholstery	sunscreen would've helped
busted ball bearings	boy and his first bike
exhausted mani-fold	yoga victim
well-built German models	thank you, Claudia
spark plug adjustment	men's hair plugs spark nothing in women
auto wreckers	auto-psy

"Hey, doc, I'd like a complete physical."

"Why?"

"Well. . . I just want a full checkup."

"But you're twenty-five years old; what exactly do I need to check?"

The fact is, a healthy twenty-five-year-old male does not need an annual physical exam, blood test, or any other screening test, other than an occasional blood pressure check every couple of years. A twenty-five-year-old female need only be seen for a Pap; otherwise she, too, is exempt from annual periodic health exams.

Older cars need periodic exams, according to the notices I get in the mail every three weeks. How often does a patient need a complete check-over? The answer depends on age, sex of vehicle, and condition. Some younger folks who tend to be a little tailpipe-retentive request exams every year. To the worried, well, I say that this is really not necessary. But as we begin to get a little rust on our bumpers and our warranties warn us they are starting to get worn, we need to be sure we are tested and screened as follows:

- Cholesterol tests every five years.
- Diabetes test every three years after age forty-five.
- Annual mammogram, fecal occult blood test, and prostate tests after age fifty.
- Eye exams every two years after age sixty-five.
- Baseline physical exam at age fifty.

Of course, should your vehicle be at risk for any particular conditions, including diabetes; prostate, breast, and colon cancer; osteoporosis; and all of the obesity-, smoking-, or sedentary-related risks, then screening and testing needs to start much earlier.

Only after these are checked, cleaned, lubricated, and back on the road can you slip into overdrive and start tooting your horn.

TOP TEN REASONS YOU VISIT US
Got a call from my financial advisors, Downward Trend.

"Dr. Dave, This is Ben Krupt," spoke a voice that immediately raised goosepimples on my goosepimples and shivered me timbers. But this time, rather than recommending I invest heavily in Enron or the California Golden Seals, I was instead asked for some advice.

"Doc, what are you prescribing for your patients these days?"

"Cyanide. You need a script?"

"Seriously, we want to know why people usually go to a doctor and what are the most commonly prescribed medications for each problem."

And so, for forty bucks, I gave him a list.

10. Hyperlipidemia, as in high cholesterol, as in high risk of heart attacks, as in high use of restaurants with "Hi, supersize that?" greetings. To determine your lipid levels, either visit your doctor or try the Jay Leno technique: "Go to the trash can, open it up, and count the number of pizza boxes from Domino's. Now

multiply by fifty." Astonishingly, the overall number-one pre-scribed drug in North America is atorvastatin, a cholesterol-low-ering medication.

9. Acute bronchitis. Nothing cute about coughing great gobs of green, gluey, frothy, fetid phlegm, courtesy of the Marlboro Man. Clarithromycin is the most popular antibiotic for bronchitis.

8. Otitis media. Blame the media for the eighth-commonest visit to the clinic. Media, as in middle, as in middle-ear infection. Unfortunately, amoxicillin is prescribed to 81 per cent of ear infection victims in North America, while in Europe antibiotics are seldom if ever used for ear infections. Kids successfully fight the infection themselves 90 per cent of the time, with a little help from Tylenol.

7. Normal pregnancy supervision, which is one of the few times people actually look forward to seeing a doctor. "I have some good news for you, Mrs. Bloggins." "Actually, it's Miss." "Then I have some bad news for you, Miss Bloggins." The commonest "drug" recommended on this visit is folic acid, a vitamin.

6. Anxiety, which is on the rise. Most sufferers are victims of fre-quent calls from financial advisors. Lorazepam is the most com-mon drug used to treat anxiety.

5. Acute upper respiratory infection, a.k.a. "a cold." Apparently, many of you suspect that your doctor has secretly developed a cure for the cold and has simply forgotten to inform the press and Nobel committees, though he must be willing to share it with you. Please don't pester us with a common cold, as it only means that we will catch your cold and spread it to our family, who will in turn curse us for being a doctor who brings home assorted communicable diseases. Surprisingly, a whopping 48 per cent of those who see a doctor for a cold manage to wran-gle an antibiotic prescription. Though it does nothing for the cold, it's often easier for the doctor to give you a drug than take the time to convince you that you don't need one.

4. Health checkups for the worried well—the routine "I am well, but I need a checkup." Twenty-five per cent of those who come

for "annual" exams don't need them. If you are younger than forty, don't darken our door, for a "routine" physical exam for no reason, Pap exams excluded.

3. Diabetes, which is a real up-and-comer as the population gets wide and fatter. Glucophage is the favorite drug used to treat this sweet sickness.

2. Depression. A real downer to see this one up there. Paroxetine, a big sister of Prozac, is currently the top prescribed antidepressant.

And the most common reason a patient will darken the door of the dear doctor is...

1. High blood pressure (hypertension), by more than twice its nearest competitor, depression! To deflate the burgeoning blood barometer, Ramipril is the top-selling antihypertensive.

"Thanks, doc, just for that I'll give you a stock tip so hot it has to eat jalapeños to cool off. Sell the farm and invest in a new company we think should do well. It's called Swimwear de Kabul."

MEDICAL MATH

Helping my son with his twelfth grade math. Since I have a science degree, it should be easy to fix these number problems, sort of like fixing my tax calculations and golf scores.

Son (starting off the conversation as he does every discussion): "Don't ever put me in one of your stupid medical columns."

Dr. D: "As if, whatever."

Son: "Okay, dad, according to this quadratic equation, the average wing speed of the swallow is what?"

Dr. D: "Is that an African or European swallow?" (Thank you, Monty.) "Now, quad means four, right?"

Son: "Good night, Dad."

Dr. D: "Good night, Stewart."

Knowing the tendency that humans have to exaggerate ("Me? Harvard, summa cum laude and about $650,000 per year"), doctors have been trained to perform integral calculus equations on any answer you give us that requires a number.

"Do you drink?"

"Socially."

"And how social are you?"

"That's a personal question."

"They are all going to be personal questions. That's why you are sitting there naked as a rat embryo. So, how much do you drink?"

"Six or seven a week."

"Beers?"

"Days."

"And how much do you consume per week?"

"About twelve beer. Less if there is no football, including arena football and soccer."

Translated: twenty-four beers.

"AND WHAT IS your weight?"

"About an hour and forty-five minutes, but hey, for your office that was quick."

"Okay, when you step on the scales, what do they say?"

"Get off! But I think I weigh about 240 pounds."

"Oh, wait, I see the nurse has already weighed you. 255 pounds."

"Well, these socks are extra thick, and I had a bunch of lint in my navel. At home, naked and with the lights off, I give myself 240, give or take a few."

"HOW OFTEN are you up in the night to go to the bathroom, Bloggins?"

"I'd say seven."

"Well, we'd better check that prostate, then."

"Errrr, ummm, 7:00 AM. I . . . I get up at seven o'clock. Other than that, I sleep like a senator."

"BLOGGINS, do you realize that gum disease has been associated with heart disease?"

"I don't chew gum no more. Can't without my teeth."

"How often do you floss?"

"Floss?"

"Forget it."

"I'VE BEEN coughing for a month, doc."

"Do you smoke?"

"Nope, quit."

"When?"

"Can't remember, exactly."

"Try."

"Okay. Maybe two o'clock, two-thirty."

(You'd be surprised how often we actually hear this one.)

"DO YOU exercise?"

"You bet, I get a real sweat going and my heart rate gets right up there for about thirty minutes every day."

"Doing what?"

"Watching *Desperate Housewives*."

"That's hardly a cardiovascular workout."

"Well, I have to find the remote first, and lifting three couches is not as easy at it sounds."

"Are they heavy?"

"Depends."

"On what?"

"If it's the African or the European couch."

BÊTES NOIRES (DOCTOR)

It may surprise you to know that doctors get our most up-to-date medical knowledge from the *National Enquirer* (Man Gives Birth to Baby with Wooden Leg, Hospitalized with Splinters!), *Sports Illustrated* (swimsuit edition), and *Reader's Digest*. The "I am Joe's Pancreas, Kidney, or Ovary" series personally got me through first-year medical school. A recent issue of *Reader's Digest* discussed ten things that doctors wish they could tell you but were too diplomatic. Included were admonishments such as: call if you're canceling your appointment, wash up, be honest about taking your medications, blah blah. But nobody has ever accused me of being tactful, and in fact, few have accused me of being a doctor. And so here are ten things we doctors would really like you to know for your visit.

1. Please turn off cell phones. While listening to your heart I get alarmed when I suddenly hear a strange galloping musical techno-tonic rhythm. So before I apply the paddles to your chest, I suggest you turn off the phone. Some of you actually insist on taking calls. "Excuse me, doctor, but I should get this. Hi, snookums! Listen, I'm in with the doctor right now, and judging by his red, swollen face, he looks busy, so let's keep this to five minutes. Yes, his waiting room is full, but I guess that's why they called them 'patient', eh?"

2. Please don't tell me the color of your pill. "I need a refill for the white one, smaller than a breadbox, you know... round, I often take it with water." Perfect. Narrows it down to 38 million medications.

3. Please do tell me your symptoms, not your diagnosis. "Well, my friend and I were studying *Reader's Digest*, and I *know* we both have the rare form of Eastern Moldavian pseudohypoparathyroidism. We need a referral right away to the best specialist in town. Oh, and if you could fill out these disability papers."

4. Don't play with your tongue stud while talking. I swear I am so distracted by watching this marble flicking out at me that you

start to morph into a Komodo dragon testing the air. "So I (click-click) was wondering if you could check my (clickclickclick) ears. I keep (clickclack) hearing this strange noise when I swallow. Kind of a clicking sound."

5. Please don't turn a child's visit to a busy doctor into a field trip growth experience. "Tell the doctor what's wrong, Aniston Moon-child." Three minutes of girl playing with shoelaces. "Go on, now. Tell him when you're ready." Three minutes of silence as she explores the blood pressure cuff. "Perhaps you could tell me, Mrs. Bloggins." "No, no, just give her time." Twenty-nine minutes later: "You tell him, Mom." This is the same parent who, just before the child is about to get a vaccine, warns, "Now don't move a muscle or this will REALLY, REALLY hurt, okay, lovepuffin?"

6. Please notice those two really large earplugs called a stethoscope that I wear when I take your blood pressure or listen to your chest. I know you're talking because I can see your lips flapping and hear some muffled noise from your lungs that sounds like Chewbacca with a sinus problem.

7. Please don't try to sneak an extra patient in. "Oh, and since we're here, could you take a look at Ron's prostate? It's been acting strange lately."

8. Please don't call and ask for medication refills without giving me any information. If I had a Nortel nickel for every message on my answering machine like, "Hey, doc, it's Bill. I need a refill of my pills. Could you call that in to the pharmacy?" Okay, Bill, but what pharmacy, what drug, and I realize you are the only Bill in your family, but... who are you?

9. Don't spit into a tissue to show me (gag) just before lunch. "It's green, doc, wanna see?" "I believe you, Bloggins." "No wait, here." (Hairball choking sound.) "Thanks for the diet idea, Bloggins."

10. Don't expect me to remember your problem from three years ago. "You remember, the rash I had on my left elbow in '87. Can you give me the same thing you gave me, the white pill, kinda round... smaller than a breadbox?"

BÊTES NOIRES (PATIENT)

After I wrote a column outlining things that doctors would really like to tell you but are much too polite to, a radio station polled its audience for a list of what patients would like doctors to know. So for those patients responsible enough to respond, here is an actual list of your responses and my response to your responses.

1. Cold hands or stethoscope can be a shocker, doctor.

   Cold is an important sensation that we are actually using to test your reflexes and see just how high assorted body parts will leap, spin, and purr, patient included. So while the stethoscope-from-the-icebox may seem like a cruel joke, we are, in fact, only doing this for you and your reflexes, sort of like smacking your knee with our rubber hammer or poking your eye with a pen. Our low chuckles of evil glee are simply a coincidence.

2. How about some magazines from *this* year in the office?

   I can only speak for myself by saying that the magazines in my office are all fairly current. We have up-to-the-minute comments by President Reagan on Iran-Contra, and you can even catch up on Cassius Clay's most recent antics.

3. Bad breath simply won't do, doctor.

   As health professionals, we have to be examples of good nutrition. I realize that there might be a slight odor to such nutritious marvels as garlic, tuna, and Snickers, but what could possibly say "eat your leafy greens" better than a sprig of parsley stuck between our teeth and gums?

4. Have someone call if you're running an hour or two behind (our time is as valuable as yours).

   This is why you are called patient and we are called many other things. We'd love to phone you, but we're pretty busy chipping ice off stethoscopes.

5. It would be great if doctors could recommend some natural remedies at times, instead of just writing a prescription.

   Just last week, I recommended hemlock for Jerry Springer.

6. The walls of those little exam rooms are so thin. I'd rather not know about that next person's odd rash.

Ahhh. This is another deliberate test, specifically of your hearing. In addition, we have found that waiting times are reduced as a result of eavesdropping. By simply announcing in the next room, "Today, Bloggins, we are conducting a study on *all* patients with this new cayenne suppository, so hold still," we find we get you out of the office quick as a bunny.

7. Speaking of paper-thin, can you actually give us a gown that's more than just one-ply? How about something with a thread count! It's cold in that little room.

The catwalks of Milan are teeming with one-plies this year. Besides, if, by the time we come into the room, your core temperature hovers around, say. . . Nunavut, the stethoscope might actually feel toasty.

8. We women would like to say that a picture on the ceiling would be nice.

And cover up the skylight?

9. We want to know you're human. Put some pictures or mementos up in your examining room of your family.

". . . and these are my sons, just prior to sentencing."

10. Don't look at our charts with that "Oh, brother, not *this* person again" look on your face.

You misread us. We are really saying, "Hey, brother, knot this person again," meaning we are pleased to have you come back for more sutures.

11. And what's with all those sick people sitting in the waiting room spreading germs?!

Here I agree. I feel that the healthy ones should be in the waiting room, while the sick ones should wait down the road by the cemetery.

12. I'd rather the receptionist wasn't so loud when asking why I'm here!

I wouldn't worry about this too much. Very few people really understand the difference between herpes zoster and herpes simplex anyways.

KNOWING A LOT ABOUT A LITTLE

There are those who would be surprised to know that I went to Harvard or even that I graduated from high school, for that matter. But one day, not too far from Harvard, my car—which has a blue book value of about $324 (when the tank's full of premium)—got all hot and bothered and needed to cool down. So I went to Harvard and took a tour. What I learned from my days—er—day at Harvard was that students here are encouraged to "know something about everything and everything about something." Harvardonians may, for example, become experts on the theoretical uncertainty of Heisenberg's thirty-first principle but also take a course on, say, squirrels.

Such is true of your medical community. GPs know nothing much about everything and everything about Hush Puppies. Specialists know an awful lot about very little. Nowadays subspecialists know even more about even less. For example, a plastic surgeon may restrict his specialty to left breast reconstruction—a breastologist. An ophthalmologist may deal only in problems of the retina in diabetics between the ages of forty-four and forty-seven, and so on.

See if you can match the symptoms to the disease and then what specialist you would get to know.

1. Your pulse is fast, you are boiling hot while everyone else is in a sweater, and your eyes bug out so far you make Marty Feldman salivate.
2. Despite Atkins, Jenny Craig, and Krispy Kreme diets, you still outweigh Botswana.
3. You bruise at the touch of a louse hair—speaking of which, your husband is now being questioned about the bruises.

4. Six months since your car wreck, your lawyer advises you that your neck, back, and earlobe pain are worse.
5. After an African safari, you return home with very high fever, chills, diarrhea, and enough ivory to make the piano blush.
6. Your HDL is low, your LDL is high, and you eat nothing but grass cuttings.
7. You have no pulse and can't breathe, and your pupils are fixed and dilated (see senate).
8. You have a rash on your elbows and knees, and now the joints of your hands are smokin' and you don't smoke joints.
9. The doctor says your prostate is lumpy and your PSA is batting 1000.
10. You see floaters and spiders and haven't done mushrooms in years.

A. Malaria
B. Psoriatic arthritis
C. Morbid obesity
D. Hyperthyroidism
E. Vitreous detachment
F. Familial hyperlipidemia
G. Chronic pain syndrome
H. Prostate cancer
I. Death
J. Idiopathic thrombocytopenia

I. Radiation oncologist
II. Retinal surgeon
III. Bariatric surgeon
IV. Rheumatologist
V. Pathologist
VI. Physiatrist
VII. Hematologist
VIII. ID (infectious disease) specialist
IX. Lipidologist
X. Endocrinologist

1-D-X; 2-C-III; 3-J-VII; 4-G-VI; 5-A-VIII; 6-F-IX; 7-I-V; 8-B-IV; 9-H-I; 10-E-II

SCORE:
9–10–You are GP material
4–8–You are specialist material
0–3–Don't get sick

POINT TAKEN
Occasionally it behooves us to take inventory of just how healthy our lifestyle is. How do you score?

Realizing that donating blood actually decreases your chance of a heart attack, you:
donate blood every three months +50
while playing hockey −35
for the Rangers −99

Your LDL cholesterol is low and your HDL cholesterol is high +50
Your blood pressure is low and your hemoglobin is high +60
Your prescription medicine is unexpectedly low and your roommate is high −75

Knowing that earwax is protective, you never put anything smaller than your elbow in your ear +65
You ram Q-tips into your ear in order to extricate the wax −70
which pops out the other side −90

You have reached your ideal weight and feel like you can go head-to-head with a pro athlete +100
Your ideal athlete is Akebono, six-hundred-pound sumo master −60
You flatten him −80

You practice monogamy +85
with all your friends −75
You believe Monogamy involves putting a hotel on Baltic
Ave. −125

You have a hearty floss daily +30
You date Heidi Fleiss −30
A quivering dental hygienist gets out barbed wire and floor
sanders when you walk in −50

By improperly trimming your toes, you end up with ingrown
toenails −40
You trim your nails straight across +30
during the sermon −90

Realizing that spirituality enhances mental health, you attend
church regularly +90
The only time you go to church is to be hatched, matched,
or dispatched −30
Your first prayer in years is on the operating room table −40
as you repeat what the priest says, including the word "beg"
seventeen times −300

You ingest lots of fiber +50
The fiber is hemp −50

You have your prostate checked annually after the age
of fifty +80
You look forward to it −70
Your name is Betty −90

You have some alcohol flowing in your bloodstream −10
You have some blood flowing in your alcohol stream −80
Your coat of arms states, "Work is the curse of the drinking
class" −90

You have a wart problem –20
but now you've licked it +/-30

This book is your main source of medical information –125
The pages of this book line the cage of your budgie,
Penelope –20
who you bought from Vietnam during "some sort of
outbreak" –50

DRUG BUST

Doctor A: "George, I've decided that the hypereosinophilia etiology is iatrogenically induced by the valacyclovir used to treat
cytomegaloviral exanthem."

Doctor B: "Okay, I'll bring the caddies."

The lexicon of medicine is so vast that entire college courses
exist solely to decipher medical terminology. It is truly a language of its own, one that encompasses difficult-sounding diseases, treatments, diagnostic tests, and procedures, to say nothing
of the origins and insertions of thousands of pieces of the human
anatomy. In addition, doctors and pharmacists must learn the
names, purposes, and side effects of roughly seven kazillion
drugs, with new and improved drugs evolving every three seconds. And just to add to the confusion, each drug in fact has two
names, a proprietary name and a generic name.

Drug companies do their best to help doctors with the Her-
culean task of remembering the names of their drugs. First, they
send drug reps to the office, usually attractive men and women
who are endowed with pleasant demeanors. They possess an
above-average ability to squeeze an entire product monograph
into thirty-seven seconds once they've snagged a doctor in the
hallway. Typically it is a "Hi there, doc, I just want a moment
to tell you about our new LintOut, a-great-new-product-that-in-
head-to-head-studies-with-other-navel-lint-removal-medications-

(inhale)-was-found-by-thirty-nine-Botswanian-experts-in-the-field-to-be-more-effective-than-our-evil-competitor."

Second, drug companies have tried not to tax the overtaxed medical mind by giving drugs names that relate to the actual purpose of the drug. These drug names can mean the difference between success and failure. An Italian gene-tech company, for example, was discouraged from using the name "GenItalia," as it was felt it would likely attract the wrong crowd looking for treatment. Other actual drug name disasters, likely developed by the same marketing genius who came up with the McDonald's "McWrap," include:

· Bumex
· Urispas
· Kriplex ("... oh, and Bloggins, there are a couple of side effects to look out for")
· Widocillin ("Hey, dear, are you *positive* the doctor told me to take this stuff?")
· Nokhel
· St. John's wort (St. Peter's mole, maybe, but ...)

Can you match these drugs with their reason for living?

1. Premarin	a. the "flu pill," tames the virus
2. Elavil	b. lowers blood sugar
3. Lariam	c. treats hemorrhoids
4. Flomax	d. really BIG hemorrhoids
5. Habitrol	e. for all migraines
6. Jectofer	f. protects from coronary disease
7. Paxil	g. pregnant mare's urine hormone
8. Tamiflu	h. fast-acting enema for sailors
9. Prevacid	i. inserted estrogen ring
10. Anusol	j. an anagram of malaria (almost)
11. Anusol Plus	k. shrinks prostates, maximizes urine flow
12. Halcion	l. iron supplement given by injection
13. Migranal	m. antidepressant, gives feeling of peace

14. Rythmol   n. antidepressant, elevates mood
15. Proctofoam   o. puts out the fire of proctitis
16. Diabeta   p. prevents stomach acid problems
17. Corgard   q. regulates the beat of the heart
18. Estring   r. sleeping pill
19. Combivent   s. nicotine patch for a smoking habit
20. Fleet enema   t. an asthma combination puffer

1g; 2n; 3j; 4k; 5s; 6l; 7m; 8a; 9p; 10c; 11d; 12r; 13e; 14q; 15o; 16b; 17f; 18i; 19t; 20h

If you scored:
0–2   Urispas
3–10 a real Bumex
11–14 not bad, but Nokhel
15–20 you are an attractive person endowed with a pleasant demeanor

BACK AWAY SLOWLY FROM THE TONGUE DEPRESSORS
Pop quiz.

Hospitals and doctor's offices are great places to go and pick up:
a. neat drugs
b. diseases
c. injuries
d. nurses
e. all of the above

The answer is e, with apologies to my own nursing staff who will now likely inflict multiple injuries (if not diseases) on me, forcing me to ingest some neat drugs.

A doctor's office can be as dangerous as a bikini boutique in Baghdad. So please be aware of these hazards:

1. Tongue depressors. Though we, as kind and entertaining doctors, love to draw little faces on our used Popsicle sticks and give them to Junior, I won't soon forget the little guy who went out of

the office and fell on the tongue depressor he had between his teeth. Suddenly, more than his tongue was depressed.

2. Liquid nitrogen. Colder than a naked Neanderthal nun in a Nunavut November, LN_2 is meant to remove assorted skin blee-bies from your hide and to perform cool, eerie, smoke-spittin' Halloween tricks. Remember high school physics class when Mr. Krywzczkrwzyrschky allowed you to dip a wire, a cord, or one of Jimmy Wagstaff's appendages in it, and then shatter it on the desk? Can still happen.

3. Latex gloves. In addition to wearing these to perform office orifice exams, etc., we often get asked by wee Wesley, "Can you make a balloon face for me, doctor?" Sure, and if you're allergic to that latex glove, Wesley, I can make *you* a balloon face. Again, no longer given out as treats.

4. Sharps box. Used needles, broken vials, Madonna's bustiers are usually out of reach of the exploring fingers of those less savvy than the sharpest kids and addicts.

5. Pap drawers. Toddler Tim likes to open this drawer and grab assorted exciting toys like the duck-bill speculums and hockey-stick swabs, then promptly shut the drawer on his fingers. Doesn't typically say "ouch, Mother," but rather screams bloody murder, causing mass hysteria out in the wailing room.

6. Stirrups. We have no palominos. Need I say more?

7. Previous patients. Who knows what exotic, highly infectious disease the individual sitting in your chair in the wailing room or on the exam table had? "Doc, I notice you're wearing a quarantine suit and a gas mask. Does that have anything to do with the guy who just left with one ear and a festering, frothy fibula?"

8. The doctor himself. Infections are spread person-to-person, and that includes the doctor who comes into your room and places a stethoscope on your torso, having minutes earlier pressed it up against an abscess of a patient dying of a highly infectious Eastern Moldavian tictyphepherpdenghivcholeraebolanitis type A.

Doctors wear apparel with crevices that harbor all kinds of potential pathogens. This includes stethoscopes, SpongeBob cufflinks, and neckties. A Florida company has actually developed an antimicrobial tie for doctors! A bearded colleague of mine used to scrub his beard in the kitchen sink after every second patient. Don't forget those pristine white coats with pockets typically teeming with bacteria, fungi, swabs, parking tickets, anatomy photos, lunch leftovers, and biopsy specimens, a virtual cesspool that has been fermenting for weeks.

In fact, the less that doctors wear, the better. The British Medical Association has now asked doctors to remove "functionless clothing items," beginning with ties. I thought of trying out this concept by showing up in my thong "Moose," but after a close call with the liquid nitrogen, I decided otherwise. True, doctors tend to wear the same white coat day after day without washing it, and yes, some never remove their ties except to restrain six-year-olds or snap them at a colleague's crotch in the surgeon's dressing room.

But I can't tell you how many times my white coat has acted as a shield against blood, spit, sneezes, sputum, and vomit, some of it from patients. To say nothing of Alphagetti and sloppy joes or its use as a walking storage cabinet of assorted secret paraphernalia. But I will agree to lose the ties (I hate to have my ascot up around my neck anyways) and SpongeBob, and I will shave daily and clean my stethoscope with alcohol, even though an intoxicated stethoscope is of little use to anyone except Lindsay Lohan. But Moose... still comes out on Wednesdays.

SCAMMERS

"The pain is awful, doctor. I can't sleep, I'm in tears most of the day, and I'm taking ten Tylenol every four hours. Is there anything stronger?"

Wayne has hobbled into the office with a fiberglass cast molded about his lower leg. Each step is accompanied by an exaggerated grimace and an occasional groan. He broke his fibula two weeks ago after slipping on a wet floor at a restaurant.

"Well, Wayne, a small bone in your lower leg shouldn't be causing this much pain two weeks after breaking it."

"You have no idea of the pain, right, Susie?"

Girlfriend/accomplice Susie nods in agreement. "He just cries all the time. But we've heard that you're a really great doctor," she offers.

"Have you tried ibuprofen?" I suggest.

"Allergic to it, doc, blow up like a balloon."

It turns out, of course, that Wayne is allergic to everything on the planet other than Dilaudid, a heroin-strength narcotic worth big bucks on the street.

I used to be a trusting sort. But over the years, MD can come to mean Master Detective. An unpleasant occupational hazard in our profession is being forced to deal with scammers, the desperate frauds who try to fool doctors in order to obtain drugs. Once a trusting young doctor who believed every patient who said they were in pain was being truthful, I have become a little more skeptical. For example, when a patient states that they have a sore back, I now counter with "YOU LYING, PILL-POPPING SNAKE!" I admit my bedside manner has deteriorated, but I do get scammed less often.

Scammers have a basket full of tricks. Commonly it is the lower back scam. The scammer has familiarized himself with the symptoms of sciatica. His/her description of the symptoms is always textbook. Good scammers can even fake some of the tests. The visit of the drug seeker becomes a game, a battle between doctor and scammer.

"So, does it hurt if you bend over?"

"oww! Oh, the pain!"

"Well, it appears as though you have sciatica, which means it should feel *better* if I step on your pancreas while stretching your right earlobe toward your elbow." (You didn't realize that medicine was this much fun, did you?)

Other classic tricks include the painful rotting tooth (that never gets fixed), the old broken collarbone that juts out, or the old scar that is supposed to represent some awful, agonizing condition. Knowing that the pain associated with kidney stones could score some decent narcotics, scammers will prick their fingers in order to put blood in their urine samples.

One doctor actually enjoys scamming the scammers. Hobbling in on crutches, the scammer becomes downright giddy when he is prescribed two hundred morphine pills. As he leaves the office, he cartwheels and pirouettes all the way to the pharmacy, only to be told that the prescription is dated Feb. 30, 2021. My colleague is targeted less often now.

Scammers are always flattering and full of praise. "You are a fantastic doctor, you are so caring, and your eyes are so blue and..." I admit, I encourage this part of the game.

"Thanks, Bloggins. Say, check out these pythons I've got for biceps."

Scammers are forever accidentally dropping their previously scammed prescriptions down the sink or into the toilet. Producing a broken or wet pill bottle, they now need a refill. Toilets have seemed to develop a voracious, albeit specific, appetite for Valium and Demerol. Penicillin somehow never gets spilled.

Scammers are constantly losing their prescriptions or having purses stolen. Some will go so far as to produce a police report "proving" they were burglarized. These same people will pilfer anything not tied down in a doctor's office, from scissors to K-Y (don't ask). This is terribly inconvenient, as it means we must go to the hospital and pilfer... er... borrow new supplies.

Back to the true story of Wayne and Susie. Wayne had actually jumped out of a second-storey apartment, thinking in his cocaine-induced paranoia that the cops were at his door. Knowing he'd broken his leg, he phoned another criminally minded friend and paid him to drive to McDonald's. Wayne then poured coffee on the floor and "slipped." He successfully sued for eighty thousand dollars.

When this plot was revealed to me a couple of months later by his accomplices, I called McDonald's. The insurance investigator decided that the money was irretrievable, likely deeply invested into Wayne's nostrils. "We've been scammed before," he admits. I know the feeling.

FUTURE SHOTS

Year: 2015

Location: Doctor's office, eighth tee

Actors: Dr. Bob and Dr. Jim. (Any similarity to actual people or animals is only a coincidence; all lawsuits will be handled by the firm of Liddy, Gait, and Tsu, located on the eleventh fairway.)

DR. BOB: *Yep, vaccination really screwed up our lives. Used to make a good living being a doctor, but...*

DR. JIM: *Nobody gets sick anymore! I miss those good old days of diabetes, heart attacks, and... hey, do you remember those folks who used to get Alzheimer's?*

DR. BOB: *Nope.*

(both laugh in a doctorly manner)

TRANSGENIC MICE, not to be confused with transgendered mice (who can't decide on what type of genes to wear), are mice that have had their genes tinkered with so that they naturally develop Alzheimer's. Some of these mice, however, were given a vaccine against beta-amyloid, the nasty wee protein that forms bundles of plaques in the brain, causing Alzheimer's. The vaccine virtually destroyed the beta-amyloid, and now mice everywhere have memories like elephants. ("Hey Frank, look over there, remember that lady who passes out when I dart across the floor? Let's go!") How nice for the mice who had genes spliced and sliced and now never think twice 'cause they have a memory that would suffice an elephant on fuzzy white dice (eat your heart out, Seuss). Since this amyloid protein is of both mice and men (rats), it may be only a matter of time until we can all be successfully vaccinated against Alzheimer's.

DR. BOB: *Yep, no pneumonia, no meningitis—heck, there's hardly an infectious disease anymore where there isn't a vaccine against it. What I wouldn't give for a good case of herpes about now.*

GENITAL HERPES currently afflicts 22 per cent of the American population, but now, according to the *Herpes Journal* (yes, there is actually such a journal; "Dear, your herpes magazine is here"), vaccines are being developed for use in preventing both infection and reinfection of herpes. The only flaw in the vaccine is that, so far, it appears to work only in women, and only in women who do not have cold sores! This no doubt will prompt an immediate name change of the disease by leading feminists to "his-pes." Of course, if fewer women have herpes, then chances are good that fewer men will get it, seeing as how. . . umm.

Trials are still ongoing for other STD vaccines, but development is a long way off, so in the meantime, no sex, please.

DR. JIM: *Yep, and I used to have so much fun giving the flu shot. But now the flu vaccine comes in a nasal spray, more like a flu snort than a flu shot. We can't even inflict a little pain anymore. I hardly feel like a doctor.*

DR. BOB: *Pain and disease on the decline. Where did we go wrong? Thank goodness for smokers, or else we'd not see any cancers, either!*

SORRY, BOB, but vaccines are in clinical trials for use in both preventing and treating several different types of cancer. And—you read this phrase here first—breast cancer vaccine. Though this approach is still in its infancy, researchers are offering hope that vaccines for certain types of breast cancer will induce rejection of breast tumors as soon as they start. Combined with a foreign agent, the vaccine fools the body into thinking that the breast cancer is an invading foreigner (rather than an invading traitor) and will mount attacks against it. The newest cancer vaccine protects against the HPvirus known to cause cervical cancer. Most exciting for all you men with prostates, tests show that vaccine therapy (using vaccines to treat cancer) may also lead to a vaccination that actually prevents prostate cancer altogether.

DR. BOB: *Your shot, Jim.*

FRED AND THE FLOWERPECKERS

Every year, a three-day "Health Show" comes to my hometown, complete with every kind of serum detoxifier, orifice cleanser, and inner-magnetic-energy-detector known to man. One thing is inevitably missing at the Health Show... health professionals. While doctors, nurses, and physiotherapists are nowhere to be found, the place is crawling with body rolfers, crystal wavers, and lots of folks who seem to view doctors and science as getting in the way of real cures. Kevin Trudeau and his band of pyramid schemers are no doubt popular at events like these.

Now, before incurring the wrath of those who believe that doctors are mired in a global conspiracy with pharmaceutical companies to ruin the world, I would like to make perfectly clear the following: I am not a nature-hating, narrow-minded, pill-pushin' prescribing purveyor of pain. In fact, I like complementary medicine, especially when a patient tells me, "You are a wonderful doctor, and I love your eyes." I recommend "natural" products such as fish oil, turmeric, navel lint, and Coors Light. I have even been known to recommend natural hemlock tea and poultice of *Amanita*, often to lawyers.

I do, however, have some reservations regarding reckless rantings such as those I heard from one "practitioner" at the show who huffed that "doctors are in bed with the drug companies to suppress the emergence of natural medicines." Somebody needs a new crystal.

1. Truckers Oughta Truck

I spoke at one booth with Paul, a deckhand on a ferry, who assured me that he could cure me of migraines, snoring, vertigo, and ectopic pregnancy if I bought a twenty-dollar jar of his essential oils and opened them by my bed as I slept. I also met Nancy, an elementary school French teacher who would perform a "live blood analysis" and diagnose medical ailments ranging from molds in my blood to unhappy white cells. I could now be cured by following her treatments. Create the disease and the cure all in one expensive sitting. Total "formal" training for Nancy was five days and a weekend of watching *General Hospital*. Finally, I fenced with Fred, a fiery, fervent fellow flaunting the latest cure for ADHD (Attention Deficit Hyperactive Demons). Fred is a truck driver who had recently got into sales of this product. "We're not saying it cures cancer just yet"—he winked knowingly while holding up his concoction—"but, by gosh, I gave it to my wild sixteen-year-old kid and he's a right regular Perry Como now." Fred, keep on truckin'.

2. Antidotes by Anecdotes

Like Fred, most of the "practitioners" had experienced some event that convinced them that a certain treatment was a yet undiscovered miracle. Though most are sincere, if not somewhat overzealous, I am concerned that science is made to appear to be more of a nuisance than a necessity.

"Can you show me any randomized, double-blind cohort studies that might indicate that East Siberian ginseng (there is a preference for exotic names) will in fact allow patients to toss away their crutches?" I inquired.

"Well," comes the reply, "we don't believe in performing studies on the blind, but this stuff will clear up your rheumatizz quicker than you can say snake oil."

3. Medicine by Multi-Level Marketing

Drugs by distributors. A guy named Bob from Boise mixes a little kickapoo joy juice with a couple of secret ingredients from Granny's cupboard. He notes that his boiseberry emu juice clears up the sinus problem of his bulldog, Mewkuss. Bob calls up Renaldo from Malibu, an expert in multi-level marketing. Renaldo, knowing how gullible people can be when enticed by nature's miracle "cures," tacks on a few more anecdotal medical benefits and sets up the "business opportunity." "Not only will this alleviate your sinus congestion, chronic fatigue, and fibromyalgia (popular targets at the Show), but by becoming a distributor, you can also become independently wealthy!" Hmmmm. What if doctors practiced the same way? "Now, Mrs. Bloggins, if you enjoyed that bladder suspension, why don't you go out and find someone who you think might also benefit. I'd get to cut, and you'd get a cut. Throw in a few gallbladders and you could make diamond level in six months."

Should a patient enjoy a sugary shiatsu or a really relaxing reflexological foot massage, then I say empty your wallet and fill your boots. But despite claims to the contrary, no amount of lavender sniffing or ancient leaves of sabu flowerpecker will cure Bob's endometriosis. The slippery slope of scientific validity became more evident to me the longer I walked around the "Health Show," never once revealing that I was a doctor for fear of becoming a hambone in a herd of hungry hounds.

I'd like to reveal even more, but I'm late for my meeting with the pharmaceutical cartel. We're going over our slash-and-burn project of the Upper Amazon.

HOLLY

Be nice to MOAS. Some of you might ask, "What's an MOA?" while others might ask, "Be nice?"

MOAS, Medical Office Assistants, or Most Omnipotent Authorities, are the amazing people you first meet when walk-

ing into a doctor's office. MOAs, the office vanguards, come pack-
aged in all shapes, sizes, colors, ages, demeanors, and abilities to
answer phones, get urgent lab results, clarify doctors' instructions
("I know what he said, Mr. Bloggins, but what he really meant
was..."), appease impatient patients, appease patient patients,
appease pharmacists ("I know what he wrote, but what he really
meant was..."), book appointments, clean examining rooms,
prepare procedures, unprepare procedures, and smile, all at the
same time. I must say I work with the best MOAs anywhere, bar
none. I won't embarrass them by telling you that Elana, Yvonne,
Michelle, and Holly are irreplaceable. I mention their names
today because I appreciate them and what they do and that they
do it without EVER a whimper. So be nice to MOAs. I know some
doctors who work with MOAs who are Mean Ornery Aardvarks,
but the women who run my office are the best. (Yes, my birthday
is coming up.)

Holly is the most difficult MOA for me to work with. This
may have something to do with the fact that she knows more
about medicine than I do and keeps me so far up on my toes
that I have corns on my blisters over my corns. Or it may have to
do with the fact that patients would rather sit and chat with her
than have anything to do with me. Exuding an extraordinary
enthusiasm about sinus infections, bladder instabilities, or gallstones, she shows a real interest in the people who house these
conditions. Patients instinctively love Holly. They love her for
her genuine concern and honest attention as well as her warm,
womanly, welcoming way. I often have to break up a knee-
slapping good time, complete with reminiscences and laughter,
as I boot her out of the exam room. She might never have met
the patient before.

Holly, thirty, has supermodel looks, a perky talk-show personality, and an IQ way above her weight. She reeks of charismatic
confidence and bubbles verve, vivacity, and versatility out every
voluptuous pore. Somehow she treats each individual as though

he or she is the most important person she interacts with that day, even though I know I am the most important.

She seems to be involved in—in fact *fascinated* by—every procedure, diagnosis, and treatment option. Possessing an intimidating intellect and an ultra-keen interest, Holly has often written the diagnosis in the patient's chart before I even see the patient. "Doctor, this looks like a case of Eastern Bohemian retroviral encephalohernia blepharitis. See me and I will explain the most up-to-date treatment."

And, since the birth of her daughter, Mia, the office constantly has to hear what a bright light *she* is. Photos of Mia are posted throughout the office daily. I believe Mia is now about to complete her reading of *Gray's Anatomy* before her admission to Harvard.

Holly's insatiable thirst to gain and share knowledge finally got the best of her. She decided to pursue medical school. She's been encouraged to become an MD by patients and friends alike, all of whom recognized her intellect and burning desire. And so she said her goodbyes and left to pursue her dream in Alberta. This book, which she studied and quizzed/corrected me on, is now my tribute to her legacy.

While en route to Edmonton, Holly was killed in a car crash. Mia survived.

So in lieu of flowers, be nice to an MOA; in fact, think about being enthusiastically pleasant to everyone you deal with out there today. Holly would have wanted that. That was her world.

ON *the*

(WILD SIDE)

PLAGUED

Every year the cockles and cackles of my heart are warmed by that sensitive and touching film classic, *National Lampoon's Christmas Vacation*. My sniffling and sobbing are replaced by shock, however, when the movie is marred by a savage demonstration of gratuitous violence. From deep within the welcoming branches of a Christmas tree, an evil menace lurks. As an unsuspecting Chevy Chase separates the tree boughs, a feisty squirrel leaps from its hideout and bounds about the house as the terrified Griswolds and guests all but destroy the holiday home in an attempt to avoid this reckless rogue of a rodent. Mothers faint, men scream, the fear is palpable. Finally, Snot the dog chases the poor squirrel through the front door and straight into a *Seinfeld* episode.

How can this wee bushy-tailed guy cause Beverly D'Angelo's (drool) perfectly dysfunctional family to go so squirrelly? Perhaps Clark and crew knew only too well that squirrels carry more than their nuts in their cheeks; they just happen to be the leading cause of bubonic plague in North America!

Each year fifteen to twenty cases of bubonic plague are reported in the west, stretching from B.C. and Alberta to New

Mexico. Fleas, infected with the bacteria *Yersinia pestis*, ride around on rodents, primarily squirrels. When a flea-bearing squirrel or rat dies of the disease, the flea flees the furry fella and finds refuge in the next closest thing to rats, namely men. Fleas jump a sinking rat like rats jump a sinking ship. They land on any human who happens to handle the dead carcass of the squirrel, prairie dog, rabbit, or mouse.

"Okay, class, after our field trip to the forest, it appears that Susie caught a cold, Billy scraped his knee, and Ralph has a slight case of Black Death. How many times must you be told not to play Hacky Sack with deceased rodents!"

A few days after exposure, the patient develops the infamous "flu-like symptoms" followed by painful, swollen lymph nodes known as buboes, or to be more medically precise, booboos. The bacteria set up shop in the blood system, and the patient becomes septic. Several antibiotics can successfully combat *Yersinia*. The plague can also be directly transmitted via respiratory droplets, courtesy of a coughing cat or human. This very nasty form of plague is known as pneumonic plague.

The Black Death scourge wiped out a third of Europe so quickly (25 million people between 1337 and 1342) that victims "ate lunch with their friends and dinner with their ancestors." Prior to Europe the plague romped through Asia, killing 30 million people. In total, the bubonic plague is responsible for the demise of 137 million humans. The last significant outbreak of plague, excluding the Spice Girls, was in 1994 in India, when disaster relief workers brought so much food that soon the rat pack and fleas invaded town, killing three hundred people.

Saddam and his happy harem of hellions knew about the plague. Along with botulism, anthrax, ricin, and smallpox, bubonic plague was one of the biological consequences of a Big Iraq Attack we prepared to contend with. But it would not be the first time that this organism has been used in biological warfare. In 1346, while busy besieging a Genoese city, the Mongol attackers were plagued with the plague. Having to rid their camp of disease-riddled bodies, they catapulted their dead comrades over the walls and into the city, prompting the Genoese to flee this flying flea market as the Old Spice Girls broke into the first known rendition of "It's Raining Men, Hallelujah."

The Japanese dropped plague-infested fleas out of planes over Manchuria in the 1930s, prompting the Manchurians to sing "It's Raining Fleas, Hallelujah." But too many of the air crew actually contracted the plague, so the Japanese packed the fleas into a shell and dropped the F (flea) bomb, an act that created mass casualties and widespread terror.

I hope most terrorists would realize that bubonic plague can nowadays be treated with simple antibiotics. But just to be safe, not neurotic, I'm going to stash away some tetracycline in my emergency medical kit. . . right under my catapult.

PESTILENCE AND PETS

"There is no psychiatrist in the world like a puppy licking your face."
—Ben Williams

Beware the dawc's dawg? It now appears that doctors without border collies are safer for you, the patient, than doctors with dachshunds. If your doctor cuddles his/her/its dog/cat/eunuch, then he/she/it might well be the cause of your untimely demise. A recent study has indicated that methicillin-resistant *Staphylococcus aureus* (MRSA), the so-called superbug resistant to most antibiotics, can be passed from pets to people (i.e., doctor folk), and then on to other people (i.e., patient folk). MRSA is a lovely mutant form of *Staph aureus* that usually does nothing more than etch out a small spider-bite-like lesion on your skin. But on occasion it can get downright nasty and spread into your body, causing other adverse effects like death and zits.

Zoonosis is the transmission of diseases from animals to humans, doctors often included as human. Children are particularly susceptible, given their propensity to want to taste what the dog tasted, lick toys that the dog licked, and fling their filthy, festering fingers freely into their mouths. As Rover scores a succulent sloppy slurp on our snout and up into our sinuses, we need to ask ourselves just exactly where that tongue was three minutes earlier.

Tens of thousands of kids in North America are infected annually with roundworm parasites, the commonest zoonotic infection passed on by dogs. While most will show no evidence of this infestation, 10,000 kids a year will develop a nasty rash, and 750 per year will have their vision affected as the worm crawls into the retina. *Toxocara canis* (roundworms) infects virtually all dogs at some time. Approximately 100 per cent (give or take zero) of pooping puppies are born infected with *T. canis*, and they shed millions of eggs per day. *Toxocara* eggs exist everywhere in our environment. Enjoy your Pop-Tarts.

Fido may have *Toxocara*, but Fluffy's got toxoplasmosis. This infection courtesy of those cute but toxic kittens, may also cause no symptoms, but on occasion it can lead to brain and eye damage. It is especially important for pregnant women not to clean cat litter boxes, as toxoplasmosis can cause birth defects. While fiddling with cat feces is one way to get toxoplasmosis, greater risks of contracting this disease come from gardening (particularly if a cat was gardening there before you) or eating undercooked meat like pork, lamb, or rack of kitty.

And cats don't get off easy with just parasites. Concerns remain regarding the dreaded avian flu (H5N1, if you speak droid). Cats tend to snack on avians and have now been found to contract avian flu, shedding the virus in their feces and nasal droplets.

Here are some easy rules to help protect your family from diseases carried by house pets:

1. Wash your hands after handling your pet—especially before eating or preparing food.
2. Take special precautions if you have a weakened immune system. Never let pets lick you on the face or on an open cut or wound, never touch animal feces, and never handle an animal that has diarrhea.
3. Don't let your pet drink from toilet bowls or eat feces.
4. Cover your children's sandboxes when not in use.
5. Use a pooper scooper. You can prevent contamination by picking up feces from your yard immediately—do not let them sit. As feces breaks down, eggs form and seep into the soil. A dog or child can play in the soil and spread contamination.
6. Feed your pets cooked or prepared food—never raw meat—and provide fresh water daily.
7. Have your pet's stool sample examined by your veterinarian every six to twelve months.
8. Ask your veterinarian to place your pets on preventive flea and internal parasite medication as soon as possible after birth or adoption. Treatment and control of internal parasites should be performed at least annually by a veterinarian.

As I peck away at the computer, my own disease-delivering dog—having just noisily groomed and slurped about her nether regions—is now licking the marshmallow topping and jujube remnants from the webbing of my fingers. "Bad dog. Go lick the kids. I'm off to examine Mr. Bloggins."

THIS BITES

Recently, my son's teenage friend appeared at our door, his face and neck bruised, battered, and stitched up with so many sutures he kind of looked like a Freddy Krueger/Elvira love child. Flatly denying a bad date with a good girl, he confessed that his sweet, serene family dog, Fangslaughter, had done this to him.

He said he'd simply leaned over the lying cur (albeit while wearing his Halloween postal-worker outfit, complete with mace and strike notice) and began to playfully tease when the dog simply up and started biting his face. There was no apparent reason for this attack, though perhaps in retrospect, resting his knee on the dog's privates (true, there's nothing terribly private about a dog's privates... more like sergeants) may have prompted the Rover rampage. Now the teen is sporting a new look for Halloween.

One of the commonest reasons for a visit to the common emergency room is common bite of pets: cats, dogs, and the common armadillo.

Cats

Our feline friends are fraught with filthy, festering fangs, and should you ever get a deep puncture bite, regardless of the size, get treated. Cat fangs are so slender and sharp that they can actually pierce and infect bone with just a wee opening! Cat bites have a very high infection rate and can be quite serious. Unless it's a very superficial scrape, I treat all bites of the hands and face, as well as any other deep bites elsewhere, with antibiotics. If you're punctured, drown the wound in peroxide and head to your doctor.

If your cat is like mine, every so often it loses its sense of animal taxonomy and snuggles into your chest thinking that you're its long lost parent. My cat then begs for some cash and the keys to the car and, when denied, it snuggles up closer, revs the motor up to Harley-Davidson level, and begins kneading me with its claws. I don't move a muscle, fearing even to breathe lest those claws be tempted to rake the very skin off my bones. I become categorically catatonic for fear of a dermal catastrophe. This is usually when my son catapults into the room testing out his new 80,000-decibel air horn. The cat takes a goodly portion of my hide with it to wherever cats go to when they evaporate their freaked-out carcasses through the ceiling. For the next few days, I end up checking myself for swollen lymph nodes to see if I've developed cat scratch fever. Although not dangerous, it can be an explanation for unexplained swollen "glands" in your armpits or neck. It is also a misnomer, as there is no fever.

Dawgs

While a cat uses the more elegant deep-puncture method, dawgs prefer the crushing approach. This means that the wound is usually not as deep, and subsequently less infection ensues. My rule of thumb and fingers is that if the bite involves the hand and is deep, antibiotics are in order. Elsewhere, watch for infection very, very carefully. Knowing where my own dog's mouth has been tends to encourage me to take the pharmacy's stock of antibiotics, disinfectants, and birth control pills.

An ounce of prevention is worth a pound of stitches. Therefore, never:

1. tease a feeding dog or cat. A dog's motto: "Bite the hand that feeds you if the hand gets between me and my Kibbles 'n Bits."
2. physically break up dog fights. Try distraction by making noise and yelling, "If you don't stop right now, someone's going to get neutered."
3. pick up strays, particularly if their collar reads "Rabid Randy."
4. touch an injured animal. A guaranteed bite or your money back.
5. pick up puppies when the mother is near. Lure the mother away first by lifting the toilet lid in the next room.
6. step on your armadillo's sergeants.

MOUNTAIN DON'T

"Daaad, I've got to go. . . .oo. . . .oo."

"Put a stranglehold on it, son, we'll be there shortly."

"Daaaad, I mean right here! Right *now!*"

"Okay! Here, use this empty Mountain Dew bottle," I relent, reaching into the back seat and handing Junior a male-compatible-bladder-relief-recyclable bottle.

A few sighs and one bitter complaint (coinciding with hitting a pothole) later, this now perfectly venomous bottle is sealed up with a cap and placed gingerly beside the seat. All is well and forgotten until we pick up number-one teenage daughter. Within seconds of hopping into the car, she cracks open the Mountain Dew and, much to our horror. . . down the hatch!

To this day, our daughter not only reflexively gags and retches each time she sees a Mountain Dew ad, but until recent therapy, she hasn't bought any drink without first making the clerk drink half of it.

Now, I realize that everyone has their own family urine-mistaken-for-soda story, but I bring this one up to illustrate the everyday occurrences of a nineteenth-century doctor. Should a patient present to the doctor with symptoms consistent with diabetes, the only way a physician could test for the disease was to actually taste the urine.

The history of diabetes goes something like this:

Long ago and far away, physicians noted that ants and flies congregated about the urine of patients who were very thirsty and urinated a lot.

Early MD Galen: "Wow, there's lots of ants swimming in that vat of urine."

Early MD Josephus: "I wonder what they're doing in there?"

Galen: "The backstroke?"

Josephus (between rib-separating laughter): "Gale, you really vivisection me."

But because MDS were too busy battling bubonic plague, syphilis, and halitosis, nobody tried to actually taste the urine. Finally, in the seventeenth century, an Oxford physician named Willis discovered the sweet, sugary taste of diabetic urine.

"Hey, guys. . . over here. . . taste this."

"Yummmm, Willi. What is it, Mountain Dew?"

This was not a good day for the medical profession. It now introduced urine-tasting into the everyday life of a doctor. Many left the profession and became hangmen or wine tasters.

Medical school interviews changed. "So, young Westminster, you wish to be a physician. Are you, sir, prepared to stamp out disease, ease the burden of the ill, and... oh... I dunno... well, do you like breath mints?"

A few years later it was noted that a dog whose pancreas had been removed ran about piddling constantly, a symptom of diabetes and something that my dog does without any freakin' disease. It was recognized that something in the pancreas must offset the dreaded and invariably fatal diabetes. Enter Dr. Frederick Banting of Toronto, and his medical student, Charles Best. Now, I don't begrudge Dr. Banting his due, but it's the medical student part that bothers me. In modern times, the only difference between a med student and dog doodoo is that you don't deliberately step on dog poop. Back then, few of us won Nobel Prizes.

But apparently, in 1921, this young fellow helped Banting discover insulin in the pancreas. They quickly extracted the insulin, injected it into diabetic patients, and the effect was nothing short of miraculous. The world rejoiced and Nobel Prizes were doled out. Dogs got to keep their pancreases, and ants resorted to moving rubber trees.

Insulin, the life saver. What a sweet discovery.

HEAVY METAL

Wilson's disease is (pick one):

a. an affliction whereby empty-headed volleyballs begin to take on a persona (e.g., Paris Hilton when extra air added) when stranded on, say, a deserted island

b. an anxiety disorder caused by a blond, menacing neighbor child, perhaps named Dennis, who plagues your sanity and drives you to go all funny-page

c. a musical lesion that develops on the soul and makes you want to Pickett sometime in the midnight hour

d. a condition where excess copper accumulates in the body, causing the eyes to grow rings and the brain to make no cents

If you selected d, you are now well on your way to becoming a doctor, should you pass the handwritten essay that must be so illegible only drug-addled pharmacists can interpret it.

A genetic disease affecting more than ten thousand North Americans, Wilson's causes copious concentrates of copper to collect in our corpses, particularly in the brain and liver. One in every one hundred North Americans carries a gene that codes for Wilson's disease. If that genotype happens to meet a similar genotype at, for example, a heavy copper concert, fall in love, and get married, then they have a 50 per cent chance of having kids with full-blown Wilson's disease.

Most of us have more copper than we need (and less gold), and our bodies excrete what they don't need, but those with Wilson's disease hang on to their copper as though it were pennies from heaven. Copper accumulation in the brain leads to psychiatric diseases or neurological problems such as tremors or difficulty walking. A copper-toned ring develops around the iris, called a Kayser-Fleischer ring, named after the German doctor who discovered it, Dr. Ring. As only one in thirty thousand have Wilson's disease, it is not often thought of when a routine liver test is abnormal, but if not treated, it is fatal.

Another metal overload disease usually associated with a genetic predisposition is iron overload, a disease that may go undiagnosed for years. Whereas copper problems manifest themselves in adolescence, iron overload begins to show up in middle age, which tends to confuse my middle-aged adolescent hockey teammates, most of whom have an overload of lead, accumulated primarily in the gluteal regions. When the excess iron that has been pumping around for years in an unsuspecting host accumulates in organs and tissues like the heart, liver, pancreas, and joints, iron overload now becomes the much-more-serious hemochromatosis. More than one million North Americans flirt with hemochromatosis, many of them asymptomatic.

Symptoms of hemochromatosis begin with fatigue, painful joints, abdominal discomfort, weakness, and weight loss.

(Many of you hypochondriacs were getting excited until the weight loss thing came up, eh?) Left untreated, heart failure, arthritis, liver cancer, and diabetes can develop. This diabetes is often referred to as "bronze diabetes," given the hue of skin in hemochromatosis.

Treatment involves a phlebotomy (flea-bother-me) or blood-letting. Patients must either be bled in a clinic every so often or play hockey against my team, lead permitting.

JERKS

I am sitting in Mrs. Krongrad's eleventh-grade English class, trying not to be distracted by the massive barnacle rooted to her chin that anchors an antenna-like twenty-eight-inch hair. As she discsses the witches of *Macbeth* as though they were colleagues, I am suddenly horrified to glance down and realize that I've come to school today without getting dressed! I am sitting absolutely starkers in the middle of high school English!

Seated next to me, and looking right at me, sort of, is none other than Lillian Facey, the doe-eycd beauty I've had my eye on since reform school. Mortification turns to horrification when the buzzer goes off and the entire class stands up, all but a stark-naked me. As I attempt to corral books, scissors, and compasses off my desk and onto my lap, I note that the buzzer keeps going and going. Only after wrapping myself in the classroom wall map do I realize that 'tis the old trusty sleep-shatterer I keep on my nightstand that clangs so mercilessly.

With sheets wrapped around me, dripping in sweat, I jolt out of bed, jerk my head around, and wait for the fog to clear to see if what had transpired while I perspired was real or a dream. I'm shaken but relieved that it was only the old recurrent nightmare of teenage angst, the partially-clothed-or-worse-in-a-public-place episode. What began as a good night's sleep turned out to be anything but, just as, to millions of people, sleep can be a jolting and jerking experience.

Nocturnal leg cramps, for example, are painful spasms that ruin a night's sleep as legs seize up. A little extra calcium, magnesium, or other electrolytes may help alleviate this. Quinine, the well-known antimalarial drug, is often prescribed for these irksome nocturnal cramps.

Another annoying sleep-disturber is restless leg syndrome (RLS). This common condition typically presents as numbness, burning, or a sensation of insects or water moving deep in the leg. It is accompanied by an irresistible need to walk or move. Of course, there may in fact be a herd of bedbugs convening on your leg, perhaps enjoying a snack of peanut butter that dripped onto your thigh as you snuck a snack of peanut butter during the night. Worse yet, it might actually be water. More often, however, it is this demon RLS that can plague you for hours and that should prompt you to see your doctor, who will be prompted to rub his chin thoughtfully and let out a long "Hmmmmm," a word that doctors practice for years. (The *hmmmm* technique is a well-recognized medical tool used by physicians in order to make patients think that they are deeply sifting your problem in their minds, when in fact they've just realized that Fluffbox, the missing cat, may be the reason the dryer at home keeps shorting out.)

The doctor will make sure your RLS is not kidney disease, anemia, or an underlying neurological problem like diabetes. Assuming that all's okay, he/she will look to treat you with either an anti-Parkinsonian drug like Mirapex, or perhaps Raid.

RLS is not to be confused with myoclonic jerk, a normal occurrence that can happen just as you are nodding off. We've all experienced that sudden spasm in our legs that occurs as we are about to enter into an entertaining dream involving English teachers and hippos. Often we tend to embed a large toe into our spouse's ear, and personally, on a real good jolt I can launch Fluffbox, my fat, furry, foot-warming feline, several feet into the evening air. My current record is seven feet, three *pffffffts*, and one ceiling fan. (Of course this disturbs her own RLK [rapid leg kicking] sleep, as no doubt she is suffering that recurrent nightmare of feline angst, being stalked by a three-hundred-pound mouse while not being able to call for help due to a large hairball jammed in her vocal cords.)

This sudden limb spasm used to be called myoclonic jolt but was changed to "jerk" later, given the frequency with which this phrase was hurled by the spouse who had just been raked by a jagged toenail.

Speaking of jerks, Mrs. Krongrad has just asked me to. . . put her map back.

THE PHANTOM OF THE OPERA-TING ROOM

With a fierce wind gusting across the tarmac, we put our heads down, held onto our hats, and headed across the runway to board our aircraft. Suddenly an empty wheelchair went flying past us, hotly pursued by a distraught flight attendant. The chair flew down the runway, pulling away each time the attendant lunged for it. It was as though a joyriding airport ghost had commandeered the wheelchair and did not wish to be caught.

Although my son was bent over laughing, I was reminded of the last time I came across a phantom and a wheelchair, many years, many patients, and many honey crullers ago. I was a lowly medical student, treated with all the respect due a kumquat. I had been asked by a physiatrist (rehab specialist) to go and interview a patient. Physiatry is a specialty of medicine best described as a combination of orthopedics, rheumatology, and neurology.

Mr. Klingfelter was a double amputee who'd lost both legs to cigarettes and diabetes, a crippling, if not lethal, combination. He had not worn his prosthetics on this particular day, and as he sat in his wheelchair, I asked him why he had come to the office. I knew he knew I was new. A jovial man, he seemed pleased to introduce me to the world of amputees.

I have always been amazed at how differently people react to an infirmity. Some, like this man, prefer to laugh at their situation. "Clipped my toenails too short one day, just kept on clipping, and here I be. But today I have an awful pain in my left foot," he winced, pointing in the direction of where his left foot once was.

Knowing he was making light of his own unfortunate situation, I decided to keep up the joke. "If you could take off your shoe, I'll have a look."

". . . and my ankle is just throbbing," he went on. This jocularity was likely his way of coping.

So, dazzling him, no doubt, with my razor-sharp repartee, I countered, "Well, sir, you've got me stumped. Where exactly did you leave your foot?"

"I'm telling you," he continued, "the pain in my foot keeps me up all night, and I'm going to need something to take the edge off." This guy was hilarious.

"It appears as though you've already taken the edge off, and then some," I responded, impressed that he was able to repeatedly joke about his injury.

Suddenly, like a lemming in a conga line, I realized I'd made a big mistake. Mr. Klingfelter was not kidding.

The physiatrist, entering the room and recognizing my confusion, chuckled and explained.

"Mr. Klingfelter suffers from pain in the phantom, a tormenting condition experienced by many amputees. He feels like the lost limb is still attached, and it is often extremely painful. Some amputees actually sense their arm resting on a table, their fingers able to feel the table's texture. Others can feel their arm reaching for a glass of water or a leg about to take a step. Some can even sense their amputated hand whenever a spot on their face is touched. But an unfortunate few will experience significant pain in the lost limb. Some mistakenly call this condition phantom pain, but the pain is very real even if it occurs in a phantom limb."

As it turns out, many of us have been amputated in one form or another. Those who have had a wisdom tooth so painful it drives them to extraction may be left with throbbing near the site of the yanked molar that can last well after the swelling has dissipated. And 30 per cent of women who undergo a mastectomy can still feel the missing breast long after the operation, a sort of phantom of the opera-tion.

But these pale in comparison to the pain that plagues 10 per cent of all limb amputees.

Treatment with drugs or even surgery has not been overly successful. A more intriguing ghost-pain-buster known as Farabloc has shown some promise in treating phantom limb pain. Farabloc is a mesh fabric of nylon and steel (Lois Lane meets Superman) that is able to shield against electromagnetic fields. In some unknown way, this fabric, when wrapped around the stump or even inserted into the prosthesis, has actually been shown to reduce pain in the phantom for some amputees.

Now, if I could just get this honey cruller storage locker by my navel amputated...

SUPERSIZE CHROMOSOME 17

I have come to realize a hard truth: fine dining and lobster dinner go together about as well as my cat and vacuum cleaners. But I've always been imbued with a warm fuzzy feeling whenever I can entice my tabby, Claws, to snuggle up to ol' Power Suck before I hit the ON switch. So, sure enough, I'm in a fine dining establishment peering down at a prettily perched piece of the Pacific in the form of the above-mentioned crustacean.

Ties, tiaras, and tuxedos were the sartorial preference of this joint, yet I was handed a plastic bib and a set of nutcrackers. No crayons. Larry the lop-eyed lobster and I viewed each other suspiciously. "Call me Ishmael!" I whispered, as I lit into this disgusting denizen of the deep.

I grabbed the claw and, with a mighty crack, released that choice meat from its brittle shell, which snapped like a week-old fortune cookie that had fallen into a really big vat of liquid nitrogen while in the Gobi desert right next to a gigantic black furry Yamaha amplifier (you Pulitzer folks paying attention?), but with unfortunate results. Not only did some pent-up juice shoot straight up into my left eye, but a wee piece of shell went hurtling across the room like a cruise missile, narrowly missing a distinguished-looking woman who was sipping at her bisque. I detected a momentary look of disdain from both her and the lobster.

Unlike the bottom-feeding lobster, which can eat whatever is lying on the ocean floor—including snails, crabs, and Jimmy Hoffa—and still keep herself looking marvelous and sweet to the taste, we are what we eat, which is why many of us resemble a Whopper with a side of Frito-Lays.

Enter the amazing science of NUTRITIONAL GENOMICS.

Many diseases are caused by what we toss past our gums. How, you ask? Perhaps I'll tell you. Nutrients actually interact with our genes by binding to DNA transcription factors. Genes, of course, are responsible for putting together our proteins, including pleasant, lovely, useful proteins that do everything from deciding how many of our great-grandmother's varicose veins we inherit to how disease-free we are. But genes that are interfered with in their intricate production of proteins can start making wonky proteins that may make us sick, homely, or start watching *Wheel of Fortune*. Thus, over time, a particular diet affects gene expression of proteins. Nutritional genomics, the study of diet/gene interactions, will usher in a fascinating new era of consumer genetics. Our genes decide if a certain nutrient, e.g., Cocoa Puffs, will be okay for our particular body, or if it will, in fact, create malignant Cocoa Puffomas on our kidneys.

Imagine going into a restaurant, handing over a disk containing your genetic profile, and being given a menu of those foods that will do you no harm. It's coming. It hurts me to admit that I already know that I likely have a malignant gene for Snickers and Tootsie Rolls. So call me suicidal. Viva death by chocolate!

Yet, despite our genomes, our body can often successfully repair nutritional damage. While working as a team doctor at the 1996 Olympic Games in Atlanta, I was taken aback by the fact that there were five McDonald's restaurants set up in Olympic Village. Not only were they open twenty-four hours for the athletes' (and doctors') snacking pleasure, but everything was completely free! For seventeen days! And guess where the athletes ate. I am not making this up. I'm not allowed to. The Olympics: fueled by Coke with a side order of Quarter Pounders. Supersized for female Turkish weightlifters.

The fifty-meter backstroke was won by a guy pumped up on Happy Meals. Sadly, however, a pre-swim feast of Big Macs spelled disaster for the Equatorial Guinean swimmer (of Sydney fame) who sunk to the bottom of the pool and ended up doing his best impression of. . . a lobster.

EATING ODDLY

"Am I fat?" Pete asked, his five-foot-eleven, 438-pound plumpness perched delicately on my office chair. "I mean, I know I'm big, but I was watching a Maury Povich show where all of these 350-pound fat folks were waddling about, and frankly, they were disgusting. I just don't see myself like that."

"I'm sooooo fat," whined Cindy, who at seventeen years of age is 108 pounds and five-foot-eight, and cannot be convinced that she is not obese.

While these two patients seemingly represent opposite ends of some psychiatric spectrum, both suffer from the same problem: eating disorders. Their distorted body images remind me of how as a kid I would pose in front of a Fall Fair funhouse mirror, bursts of compressed air shooting out the floor and up my pant leg, frightening my nether regions into hibernation. I'd marvel at the odd distortions the mirror reflected back at me, shapes that, now that I've reached middle age, occur in regular mirrors.

Pete suffers from so-called "night-eating syndrome." He doesn't actually eat the night, but if the moon hit his eye like a big pizza pie, he'd down it. He rarely eats breakfast but crams in more than half his daily calories *after* dinner. He grazes on carbohydrates throughout the evening and even wakes up to eat during the night. Despite feeling guilty the next morning, he repeats this pattern night after night, becoming increasingly anxious, upset, and depressed. A whopping 27 per cent of those who are one hundred pounds overweight eat this way. The fact that they eat mostly sugars, which can stimulate "feel-good" neurochemicals, has led researchers to believe that these people may be self-medicating mood disorders.

Night-eating syndrome is not to be confused with nocturnal sleep-related eating disorder (NSRED). How often have you been awakened in the morning by the dog licking chocolate mousse off your face? Ever woken with a half-eaten tomato-and-soap sandwich perched on your pillow? If so, either you may suffer from NSRED, or your dog may be having a little prankster fun at your expense. Sufferers of NSRED sleepwalk and sleep-eat. Part of their brain is sleeping while the very large area of the brain responsible for Snickers and the like is wide awake and screaming at the top of its neurons, "Suuuuuueeey!" High-fat comfort food is the object of their midnight missions, food that they may be restricting themselves from eating during the day. Occasionally they get confused and end up slicing soap instead of cheese, or thinking they are munching peanuts when they're actually enjoying a handful of Kibbles 'n Bits. (This greatly perturbs the dog who, in a huff, heads to the kitchen looking for tomatoes.)

Cindy, with anorexia nervosa, somehow perceives her body to be that of Pete's. Anorexia can be an extremely difficult disorder to treat; the cause of this illness that creates bony, brittle bodies still remains a mystery. Often anorexics are self-critical, over-achieving perfectionists who have a weight-gain phobia so severe that the thought of an extra pound will provoke them into an extra pounding of their body. Using laxatives, excessive exercise, and bulimia, they eventually destroy their bodies and minds, sometimes with fatal consequences.

Another intriguing eating disorder you'd hate to discover in your family tree is pica, from the Latin for "magpie." Those who have pica actually eat dirt, paint chips, coffee grounds, ashtray contents, rust, cornstarch, baking soda, soap, and other items not usually considered food outside of a college dorm. As many as 15 per cent of children may suffer from pica, as do a hefty proportion of pregnant women. Pica sufferers may have an underlying mineral deficiency such as iron, or they may just be nuts.

While eating rust and ashtray contents may appall you, how many people do you know who still smoke?

One more. Orthorexia nervosa is a term coined to describe those who are fixated on eating superior or pure food. They feel superior to those who eat from regular grocery stores. Their food comes from the best sources, and they often consider health food stores their only option. They obsess over what to eat, how to prepare it, and where to procure the premium food. Eating the best food becomes more important to their well-being than anything else, including relationships, career, money, and even hockey.

Can you imagine the offspring of a pica and an orthorexic? "Okay, kids, eat up your pure free-range antibiotic-free tofude-beast, bred on the moors of East Elbow, England. For dessert, Daddy is going to share with you whatever is stuck on his shoe."

GOOD TO THE LAST DROP

To teach my eager troop of Boy Scouts a thing or two about civic responsibility, I decided to change this Thursday evening's activity from "creating pipe bombs from chipmunk poop" into "a trip to the blood bank." Wide-eyed (a fear response all Boy Scout leaders live for), the boys filed into the blood bank to learn why every responsible healthy adult should donate blood and how that could possibly include their leader. With one squeamish eye on the needle entering my arm and the other on the cookies and juice table, my intrepid Scouts gawked as a unit (one pint) of red liquid gold was mined from my vein.

"Any questions, boys?" asked the nurse, who, much to the surprise of the scouts, did not have oversized fangs or sound like Ivana Trump.

"Yes, where's the washroom?" came the first urgent inquiry from a wobbly Scout who looked more apt to barf than snarf cookies.

"Who uses the blood?"

"Blood can be stored for only forty-two days. We need fifty thousand units every day in North America. All of us, at some time, will either need blood or have a family member who needs blood." The nurse went on to give the surprising statistics of who needed blood the most:

- car accidents   four to six units
- brain aneurysm   four units
- hip replacement   two units
- heart bypass   one to six units

Rangers game:

- goalie   eight units
- defenceman   twelve units
- fan   thirty-six units

"Can I give blood?"

"Nope. You must be between seventeen and seventy-one and healthy. After age seventy-one you buy your own cookies."

In order for blood to be safe, you can't give blood if you've been to the dentist in the past three days (three months after my dentist), had a tattoo or piercing in the past twelve months, or even if you have a cold. Those who can NEVER donate blood include those who have used IV drugs; or have had hepatitis, HIV or cancer; or have been engaged in homosexual sex, paid for sex, lived in the Bronx, or dated George Clooney. Millions of us could donate blood, but less than 5 per cent of eligible adults actually do. And isn't it usually the same people who never donate blood who are the first to complain when none is available for a surgery? Lack of blood means cancellations of surgeries or worse yet, play-off games.

"Are there any benefits to me to donate blood?"

"In fact, there are," the nurse replied:

"1. You get a cool sticker.
2. At the time of donation you are screened for anemia, cholesterol, and several blood-borne infections.
3. It is quite possibly good for your own health. For those who need a less-than-altruistic reason to donate blood, there may, in fact, be some personal benefits. Some studies, currently in the process of being reproduced, have shown that men who donate blood annually suffer 88 per cent fewer heart attacks than non-donors. It has been postulated that ridding ourselves of old iron-heavy blood and stimulating new blood might decrease heart disease. (Women's routine monthly bleed may be one reason they live longer; the other is that they don't ride bikes with horizontal top tubes.)
4. You get Oreos every Tuesday."

"Do you have a motto that could motivate the public to donate blood?"

"We're trying to decide," the nurse responded. "We've narrowed it down to four:

IT'S IN YOU TO GIVE.

WE NEED YOUR TYPE.

GOOD TO THE LAST DROP.

HURTS LESS THAN A SPINAL TAP."

PERSONALITY TRAIT . . . OR DISORDER

"Carl," I comment to the psychiatrist sitting beside me at a medical conference I recently attended (for some odd reason, these guys seem to relish sitting by me), "is it not true that just about everyone could be slotted into one personality disorder category or another?"

"Sort of. We could all be described as having one style of personality or another, with only the degree of the personality trait determining if it becomes a disorder. You, for example, I would classify as a compulsive personality with a touch of narcissistic. . ."

"Why, you incompetent, Freudian, snake-oil nincompoo. . ."

"No, this is true of most doctors. But a personality style only becomes a disorder when it is taken to the extreme. Then it begins to interfere with day-to-day functioning. But, by its very definition, those with personality disorders don't believe they have a problem. They think they are okay; it's everyone around them that notices the problem."

"Funny, I've noticed that my entire office staff, my hockey team, and my family all seem to have problematic personality disorders."

"I see. While 2 to 3 per cent of the population consistently demonstrate a full-blown personality disorder, the rest of us need to be wary that our particular personality style doesn't deteriorate down the continuum into a personality disorder. Certain triggers, such as an illness (particularly neurological illnesses), stress, and even some medications may convert our style or trait into a disorder. For example, someone you might consider 'sensitive' may become ill and slide down that continuum to develop an avoidant personality disorder. A 'conscientious' person may become an obsessive-compulsive during university exams.

"While personality traits are often genetically programmed, a dysfunctional personality disorder may develop permanently in a child who is the product of chronic moderate neglect or abuse. Once ingrained, personality disorders are notoriously difficult to treat. It is not easy to treat someone who thinks everyone else is the problem. These people are able to thwart any attempt at therapy. They are 'difficult' people with disturbed, extreme, and rigid views of themselves and the world about them."

Want to get the family stirred up tonight? Try gathering the clan around and determine which personality trait/style each fits into. That way, when Uncle Archibald goes squirrelly one day while on Demerol after bowel surgery, you can predict which personality disorder you will be dealing with.

To further foment family feuding, grade each player from one to ten based on how close their trait is to becoming a disorder.

PERSONALITY STYLE	DISORDER
vigilant	paranoid (unwarranted suspicion, envy, distrust in motives of others)
devoted	dependent (submissive and clinging behavior, fear of separation)
mercurial	borderline (very unstable in interpersonal relationships, impulsive)
self-confident	narcissistic (lack of empathy for others, need for admiration)
dramatic	histrionic (overreactive, theatrical behavior and seductiveness, attention-seeking, excessively emotional)
aggressive	explosive (impulse control, temper problems)
adventurous	antisocial (disregard for rights of others, sociopathic)
conscientious	obsessive-compulsive (excessive concern with conformity, inability to relax easily)

PERSONALITY STYLE	DISORDER
solitary	schizoid (timidness, introversion, social detachment)
leisurely	passive-aggressive (negativism, passive resistance to demands and responsibilities)
sensitive	avoidant (hypersensitive, social inhibition)
self-sacrificing	self-defeating ("If I suffer enough and someone sees it, I'll be loved")
idiosyncratic	schizotypal (eccentricity of behavior, discomfort with and reduced capacity for close relationships)

Once the game is over, surviving family members may decide to play something safer next time, like Hungry Hippos or Russian Roulette, or perhaps create a new game like Pin the Tail on the Carl.

SLIMY SURGEONS

WARNING: *NOT TO BE READ AT DINNER TABLE* (or in vicinity of sushi, white rice, or sensitive leeches)

"Forceps, stat!"

"Here you go, doctor."

"Hemostat, stat!"

"Yessir."

"Stats, stat!"

"The Leafs are three points up with a game in hand and. . ."

"No, no, the patient's vital stats."

"Pulse is thirty, respirations eighty-nine, and her mutual funds are at 18.9 per cent."

"That's better. Now leeches, stat!"

"Leeches, sir? Don't you think that maggots would be more appropriate here?"

Among the seething whirls and whistles of high-tech hospital lasers, fiber optics, and designer bedpans rests a simple aquarium crawling in leeches. Leeches have slithered back into our hospitals, now with a meaningful job to do. These slimy surgeons sit back in their little leechy surgeon's lounge, smoke cigarettes, and discuss recent cases, recent wives, and politics (kindred spirits). Occasionally they perk right up, hopping up and down madly and wagging their tails with anticipation every time a plastic surgeon happens to walk by the aquarium.

Plastic surgery is what they do best. A day in the OR for the leech means a succulent feast of blood. They utilize their three hundred teeth and a unique ability to inject an anti-clotting agent in order to suck up undesired engorged blood from re-attached fingertips, earlobes, lips, and even tongues. If too much blood is left in these reattached pieces, then the congestion may cause the tissue to die. Leeches are even being used to treat the congested blood of hemorrhoids. ("Good news, Bloggins, that massive barnacle in your behind is now fully decompressed; bad news is WE CAN'T FIND THE LEECH!")

The hospital actually buys the leeches, at about eight dollars each, from the tax department, where they are bred en masse. The leech wrangler—a nurse, usually named Sarge—can get pretty "attached" to the little surgeons. She gives them names such as Robin Leech (prefers blue blood), F. Leech Bailey (according to my lawyer I should make no comment here), and Pamela Anderson Leech (definitely no comment).

After a forty-five-minute fling in the OR, however, the leech, now stuffed to its gills, is classified as biohazardous waste and is therefore sent to the hospital cafeteria. Not only do the leeches perform the surgery, but they also provide their own anesthesia. As any schoolboy—who, on a sunny afternoon, has substituted math class for a day of searching out swamp frogs and crawfish—knows, the leech attachment is pleasantly painless. Exiting the swamp covered in painless leeches, frog in one hand and blood dripping down the legs, is a joy that only a child of the male species would understand.

If the leech on your tongue idea hasn't put goosebumps on your goosebumps yet, perhaps a doctor at the foot of your bed barking, "This patient needs a new dressing, and throw some maggots on that wound, will ya?" might convince you that you're a guest of the Addams Family Memorial Hospital. In fact, these cuddly little botfly babies are also making a comeback in some hospitals. Prior to the introduction of antibiotics in the 1940s, some three hundred U.S. hospitals used MDT, or maggot debridement therapy (debridement meaning your wife leaves you should you ever incur this treatment).

Any dead tissue sitting in a wound is a serious source of infection. To maggots, it's a smorgasbord. Doctors noticed that soldiers' wounds were cleaner and healed better when infested with maggots. These patients required less nursing care (nurses refused to go near them), and wounds healed better. As antibiotic resistance develops at an alarming rate, Maggie the Maggot is once again in vogue and is actually being used in some hospitals to clean out bedsores, diabetic foot wounds, post-op wounds, and skin ulcers.

The future may hold more interesting biotherapy, including slugs to treat depression, mussels for muscles, and hornets for impotence. It fact, it's sunny out right now, and in the interest of medical research. . . I think I'm gonna put my hip waders on.

SCAB LABOR

I am a pretty picky picker. In late summer in my town I head out to pluck the plumpest, purplest, perfectest blackberries in town, a masochistic exercise known to its practitioners/victims as pick and prick. In August, the blackberry-picker's chant can be heard resonating throughout the valleys for many miles. "Mmmmmm, OUCH!, mmmmmm, CRAP!, mmmmmm, WASP!" (Repeat.) I'm protective of my favorite spot, and if I happen to see anyone picking in the very area that I intend to pillage, I point them to the freshly posted signs that read "Bubonic Plague Zone" or "Medical Parking Only." If that fails, then I subtly torch their car.

Once picking, I am never happy with the berry I have just picked/squashed. I glimpse that prize berry just beyond my reach. Like a bear sticking its bare snout into in a busy beehive, I extend myself fully to nab it but get viciously snagged by several lesser, jealous berry branches. My hands become a patchwork of deep purple berry juice and deep red hemoglobin. Ahhh, the joy! Ohhh, the pain!

Later in the fall, I pick mushrooms, keeping in mind at all times the old adage: "You can be a bold mushroom picker or an old mushroom picker, but you can never be both."

But many pickers are not seasonal pickers. They live in their own skin all year long, and it seems to say to them, "Pick me, pick me!"

Twenty-seven-year-old Julie had more scabs than a labor strike, more scars than Michael Jackson, and more stress than a snake crossing the track at the Indy 500. Her face, scalp, shins, and the parts of her back that she could actually reach had been scraped and picked over like a dead varmint in Vultureville. Some scabs were infected and had become very itchy. With great medical acumen I surmised that she simply couldn't help herself, after she said to me, "Doctor, I simply can't help myself."

Julie suffers from neurotic excoriations (NE), an unfortunate yet common picking disease of the skin. Like all impulse control disorders, tension builds up and the impulse to pick becomes uncontrollable. Julie experiences momentary relief as she heads to the mirror and picks out imaginary threads, but this is soon followed by shame and guilt as tears flow and mingle with the blood on her over-picked, undermined face. She repeats this several times a day and has actually been placed on disability because of it.

NE can be a manifestation of stress or a symptom of an underlying psychiatric disease such as obsessive-compulsive disorder, depression, or borderline personality disorder and self-mutilation.

I have a long, spindly wooden back scratcher sitting on my desk right next to Gumby and Pokey. I call him Handy. He is the finest piece of sculpture in my home and one of my best friends. He has five reliable wooden fingers that never complain when I send him down the back of my shirt to do a task that only a wooden hand could love. In fact, I am scratching at this very moment as I type with my nose.

Like most men and beasts, I love a good scratch. If Handy goes missing, I get quite upset and throttle my sons until he reappears, usually where I left him in the bathroom (don't ask). Am I abnormal? Perhaps, but not because of my scratching. Scratching becomes pathological when it goes on for hours, forming cuts that never heal as they are picked, scratched, and rubbed again and again. Many over-scratched victims cover the damage with makeup; others don't leave home because of it.

But now there is good news in this battle against problematic skin picking. Julie was placed on an SSRI medication, and in a very short time she has responded dramatically, though she still succumbs to the pick urge on occasion. She now needs no extra makeup other than to cover some old scars, and she is functioning normally. She works full-time and has taken up new hobbies, including cycling, knitting, and baking homemade pies. I provide her with the berries.

LIGHTING UP

It was painfully obvious that thirty-four-year-old Tammy had incurred a nasty sunburn, given the shiny, blistering face that greeted me as I entered the treatment room. But this burn, unlike the ones usually seen the first super sun-soaked Saturday of summer, had a very bizarre pattern. The redness and blistering was elliptical, surrounding the middle of her face but leaving the outer parts white and untouched. It looked as if she'd worn a snorkeling mask filled with acid.

"This burn really hurts, doctor, and I need to know if there will be any scarring," she pleaded apologetically.

"How exactly did you get this?" I inquired.

"Well, don't laugh, but. . ." (Note to patients: Warning a doctor not to laugh at the absurd explanation you are about to offer induces a sudden clenching of most sphincters, accompanied by a look of forced seriousness with furrowed brow and clasped hands. The doctor seldom speaks, given the fact that he is biting the insides of his cheeks to keep from bursting out in hysterics.)

". . . I read that sunlight is good for depression, so I stuck a sunlamp on my face."

Another hapless victim of myth information. I wondered if this was meant to cure or cause her depression.

Years ago, when my family moved from the city to the country, we decided that to keep up with the Clampetts, we would raise us some chickens. That fall we built a pen, bought some hens, and waited for the eggstravaganza. But nothing. The chickens just strutted about looking ridiculous. I called a local henologist, who advised me that chickens need a certain amount of light before they start laying and that I should quit calling them names and making wringing motions with my hands. Sure enough, as the days got longer that spring, eggs galore, much to the pleasure of my sons and the chagrin of local bus and school windows.

To 10 per cent of the population who live in northern climes, shorter days mean longer faces. Seasonal affective disorder syndrome (SADS) is a type of depression that begins in the fall and lasts through winter (see Maple Leaf fan). SADS presents as an atypical depression. Where good old-fashioned run-of-the-mill depression usually means sleeplessness and anorexia, the SADS variety of depression will have its victims overeating, oversleeping, craving carbohydrates, and gaining weight. Autumn angst and winter woes may also bring increased interpersonal conflicts and even lower resistance to infection. Some children may have more significant behavior problems in the fall and winter.

Bright light, sent to the brain via the eyes, modifies serotonin, a neurotransmitter well known to play a major role in depression, mood, and possibly beer. Light also affects production of melatonin, a hormone made in a small light-sensitive spot under the brain known as the pineal gland. Melatonin initiates and maintains sleep. Elderly insomniacs produce little melatonin, a situation made worse by the poor lighting in some institutions. One fascinating study showed that supplemental bright light, given for four hours during the day, reversed insomnia in the elderly and created what is known as the senate. Bright light resets our daily biological rhythm so that more melatonin is manufactured at night.

SADS is so common a condition that almost all university hospitals in the northern half of North America have a SAD clinic, complete with SAD nurses and SAD doctors. The mainstay of treatment involves supplemental light, not an unfiltered sunlamp. Forty-five minutes of bright light (10,000 lux) each morning can be as effective as Prozac. In fact, combining light therapy with Prozac or a similar drug can dramatically reverse depression in less than a week. Sitting and reading twenty inches away from a white fluorescent light placed at a forty-five-degree angle allows the eyes to pick up the light and redirect it to the light-starved brain. Should you need to lighten up your day, light boxes can be rented or purchased. It would be wise to first talk to a SAD doctor in order to confirm the diagnosis. Do not fry your face with a sunlamp. Light therapy is now also being used for PMS, bulimia, and jetlag and studied for post partum depression.

So, whether you're a chicken who's been egged on to produce or you eat and hibernate too much each winter, see your vet/ doctor, and just maybe... we'll leave the light on for ya.

TV TURNOFF

Serena, a perky ten-year-old figure skater, was brought in to the clinic by her dad. She had injured her left leg while skating and was wondering if she might have broken a bone in her shin. I asked her to hop up as high as she could and to land on the injured leg because, well, I have a bit of a mean streak. Besides, if the pain is worse on landing than on takeoff, then there may indeed be a fracture.

Serena flashed her pearly whites at me and hopped way up on her left leg but came down on her right leg. As she landed with her arms spread open, she leaned forward, arched her back, and smiled a huge grin for the French judge. When I explained that I needed her to try to land on the same leg she jumped from, she tried again. But again, she landed on her right leg, smile intact. Her father, a little embarrassed and concerned that she'd whacked her noodle one time too many on the end boards, explained to her what she was to do. Again and again, whenever she jumped off her left leg, she would reflexively land on her right, accompanied by a large swoop with her arms. This was how she was trained. Her habit had become pure reflex.

PAVLOV'S DOGS would salivate whenever they heard a dinner bell ring. (My dogs salivated whenever they breathed.) Most of us are hapless creatures of habit, no different than Serena's skates or Pavlov's puppies. But our habits eventually become reflex.

THE LAST WEEK in April has been designated National TV Turn-off week. This might explain why nine months later we celebrate National Obstetric Week, which may explain why another week after that is National Don't-Ever-Come-Near-Me-Again Week. While I appreciate the efforts of this Washington, D.C.–based organization to want to help change a TV habit that has become overwhelmingly destructive to both our physical and mental health, I would recommend two things. First, change the focus to National TV Turnoff YEAR, and second, don't you people know that the last week in April is smack in the middle of the Stanley Cup play-offs? That's like telling a spring rabbit it's National Celibacy Week or a great white shark it's National Vegetarian Week.

A father of two Olympians in my community was once asked how he had two children who became Olympic athletes in two very different sports. His answer: "We got rid of our TV."

Breaking the TV habit would free up 28 hours a week for the average adult (228 hours a week during the play-offs) and 21 hours for the average kid.

Watching TV is not only habit-forming; it can also determine what habits our children develop. A study out of Dartmouth Medical School showed that 46 per cent of children who were allowed to watch whatever they wanted had used alcohol by the eigth grade. Those who had strict restrictions in their movie-viewing had a different outcome, with only 4 per cent drinking alcohol. The same was true of smoking, 33 per cent to 2 per cent. Only 16 per cent of kids in the study were *not* allowed to watch R-rated movies. Astonishing! To you parents of those 16 per cent I say, well done. You are thoughtful parents. You might have saved your children from developing habits that ultimately could land them in doctor's offices. By monitoring or turning off the TV, you are helping to create more of society's Doers rather than life's Watchers.

I challenge you, for your children's sake, to do something remarkable and deep-six the boob tube. You may need to load up on Prozac and wait until after the play-offs. But without the TV, you'll share games rather than game shows, thoughts rather than thoughtless TV treacle, and time with your family and friends rather than wasted time. Reality shows will be replaced with reality. Entertainment may be real, lively, and interactive rather than experienced vicariously from a couch.

So take a deep breath and YANK that cable. Now go out and land on the other foot.

BETHUNE

In a brave annual quest to undertake two new challenging experiences, I decided this year to learn to speak Mandarin and to
have my teeth cleaned—both of which, I have discovered, emit
similar sounds. Planning to go to China to practice medicine for
a month, I knew it might be wise to brush up on the language.
I have nightmares of accidentally insulting the wife of the chief
executioner by suggesting that she resembles the southern
exposure of a northbound Pekingese and gives off the odor of a
rancid yak.

What makes learning Mandarin tough is that the same word
can mean several different things, depending on the intonation
used. "Mei" can be *mei*, or simply mei. If spoken as though a
sensitive part of the male anatomy has just been caught in a
Cuisinart, then "mei" means "buy." If the exact same word is
spoken with the intonation of Deputy Dawg on helium, then
it actually means "sell"! I believe my financial advisor was woe-
fully unaware of this when he invested heavily for me in Far East
markets.

In order to practice my new lingo, I took my skills to a local
Chinese restaurant, figuring I could converse courageously with
phrases like, "I am pinhead. You have nice kangaroo." My first
attempt to speak to the waitress seemed to go well until, reaching
down for a guttural intonation, I accidentally dislodged a sweet-
and-sour chicken ball, turning it into a cruise missile.

"Your accent is excellent," she winced. "Why are you going to
China?"

When I mentioned I was practicing medicine, she astonished
me by immediately invoking the name of Bethune. Remarkably,
another Chinese lady had mentioned his name to me the previous day, when I spit out my intention of going to her homeland.

Alcoholic, womanizer, egotist, cranky, Communist, twice-
divorced hero Bethune. Though he lived there only eighteen
months, he left such a powerful legacy in China that he is a

household name there even six decades after his death. The story of Dr. Norman Bethune illustrates how one man, despite many personal flaws, can influence the attitude of an entire nation toward another. To many Chinese, Canada is synonymous with the international humanitarian Bethune. Any man who gets his mug on a stamp from two countries must have been well-liked and is now well-licked.

Born at a young age in 1890 in Gravenhurst, Ontario, Henry Bethune knew what he wanted to do while still a wee lad. He so admired his surgeon grandfather, Norman, that at age eight he hung Granddad's nameplate in his bedroom and demanded to be called Norman. Injured as a stretcher-bearer and sent home early in wwi, he learned medicine and three years later returned to the same battlefield as a surgeon. In 1929 he contracted tuberculosis. "It's not the cough that sends you off," he stated, "it's the coffin they send you off in." While waiting to die in a sanatorium, he read of an experimental radical surgical procedure to treat TB, one he insisted on undertaking. Impressed with the outcome, he decided to study thoracic (chest) surgery. He invented several surgical instruments still used to this day, including rib separators and the iron intern.

Bethune rose to Chief of Thoracic Surgery in Montreal, complete with all the accolades and the wealth that accompanied that lofty lot in life. But his disillusionment at the disparity of medical treatment based on wealth turned him into a man with a mission, one that would cost him his life but make him a hero. He traveled to Russia, where he was impressed by the universality of health care. In 1936 he went to Spain to help in the fight against Franco and his fascist friends. But drinking and carousing got in the way, and he outlived his welcome. By now, he was seeing red. In 1938 the Second Sino-Japanese War beckoned him.

"I am going to China because that is where I feel the need is greatest, that is where I can be most useful," he said. He operated under shellfire. He took no pay. He shared his clothes, his food, and his blood and was never happier. He was a doctor's doctor. And when he accidentally cut his finger with a scalpel, he incurred fatal blood poisoning.

Though he had been sent a private stash of sulfa drugs that could have cured him, he had already used these up on his patients. His death prompted Mao Zedong to eulogize, "I am deeply grieved over his death. We must all learn the spirit of absolute selflessness from him. With his spirit, everyone can be very useful to the people. A man's ability may be great or small, but if he has this spirit, he is already noble-minded and pure, a man who is of value to the people."

Xie xie. (Thank you)

REEFER MEDICALNESS

What is your town's Compassion Society up to these days? Euthanizing boy bands? Sterilizing mosquitoes? Vice versa? Compassion societies are those intrepid organizations that deal in marijuana for medical use. Motto: "Hey, dude, where's my care?" Or, as one client appreciatively describes, "They put the hash in compassion."

In an effort to weed out some of the misconceptions clouding this budding market, I called the local Compassion Society and was invited to come down and check out the joint. Realizing that the location of the society is a well-guarded secret, my inquiry, "How do I get there?" was met with, "Use your freakin' car, man."

Knock knock knock.

"Who's there?"

"It's Dr. Dave."

"Dave's not here, man."

"No. *I'm* Dave."

"Oh, hey, man, come on in."

Expecting to enter a pad full of tie-dyed, red-eyed, dread-locked dudes lounging about making rude noises with vacuum cleaner hoses sucking away at their bottom lips (my dog freaks when I do that), I was surprised at how clinical the office was. Add some 1956 *Life* magazines, fuzzy mold, and a few screams of pain, and this could have been my own office. Each patient at this clinic had a separate chart, complete with a referral from a doctor. Marijuana is doled out but not consumed on the premises. Local MDs refer patients whose illnesses range from irritable bowel to fibromyalgia, and from glaucoma to multiple sclerosis. Most of these patients have tried prescription after prescription without success and have admitted to their doctors that the one thing that seems to give them some relief is marijuana.

In fact, marijuana has been found to be useful medication for those who suffer:

· severe nausea, often associated with chemotherapy.
· wasting diseases, including cancer and AIDS. These folks need the munchies.
· spastic conditions secondary to neurological diseases.
· chronic pain syndromes, including irritable bowel and fibromyalgia.

Some doctors fear recommending marijuana. Aside from the usual concerns of medication dosages, purity, and interactions, doctors remain somewhat averse to yanking out their script pad and scribbling, "Smoke two of these and call me in the morning" (particularly in jurisdictions where we could end up having to wear soap on a rope). As part of the MD job description, we spend no insignificant portion of our day describing in great detail how a patient will incur assorted horrible cancers of assorted horrible organs if they continue to smoke. It's then awfully awkward to instruct the next patient to "burn these leaves and inhale the smoke deeply into your lungs."

But really recent, relevant research has shown that there is, in fact, no increase in lung cancer from smoking marijuana. Furthermore, vaporizers allow the active ingredients of marijuana to be inhaled without actually burning the leaf. This college dorm invention was created to prevent telltale odors from wafting into the dean's lounge and mixing with his telltale odors.

Marijuana, like Valium and Demerol and other drugs, should *not* be used recreationally. Marijuana can render serious users seriously stupid (hence Pauly Shore). More marijuana users driving Pontiacs, dental drills, shopping carts, or other dangerous equipment is not what society needs. However, medical marijuana could be made available to those who suffer and would benefit from its use.

Having got the dope on how this growing operation works, I wished these altruistic cannabis experts good luck in their endeavor to bring relief to the discomforted.

"Thanks for checking us out, doctor. And by the way, before you leave, could you turn your pockets inside out?"

DRESSED FOR STRESS

At the end of the final year of medical school, graduating students search for a hospital that will take them on as interns. An internship ensures that the potential doctor will complete one to two years of compulsory hospital work before being turned loose on an innocent community. This is a stressful time for docs-to-be, as there are many more prospective interns than there are hospital internship positions. Applications are made, interviews are conducted, and prayers are sent heavenward.

It was at that time in my life that I learned a profound lesson about handling stress. Having ventured west to British Columbia, I had to decide between interning at a hospital in Vancouver or one in smaller, quieter Victoria. Not wanting my medical skills to get rusty, I went golfing in Victoria. While waiting for the octogenarians, who were busy octogenering on the sixth tee box, to play, I explained my predicament to one venerable veteran of Victoria who was about to tee off.

I'll never forget his response. He pointed his driver at me (which I believe was a putter). Comparing busy Vancouver to quiet Victoria, he stated that, though they were both nice places to live, the difference between living in the big frenetic city of bad sports teams and living in Victoria is that "Here, in Victoria, we don't walk up the escalators, we get on for the ride!" Right then and there, I chose Victoria.

The mind and body are as intimately connected as Bill Clinton and cigars. Should the mind be suffering too much persistent, negative stress, the body often wears it. In fact, a huge percentage of patients who visit a doctor in North America these days have medical conditions related to stress. Besides the obvious psychological difficulties, stress may cause physical illnesses such as high blood pressure, ulcers, asthma, insomnia, heart disease, PMS, herpes attacks, colitis, dental problems, arthritis, backache, numerous skin conditions, headaches, irritable bowel syndrome, and many more dis-eases, ranging from cancer to colds.

Might you develop one of these illnesses because of... stress? The following test may predict. If one of the following events listed below has occurred in the past year or is expected to occur in the near future, record the score as many times as the event has or will occur this year. For example, if you get divorced, remarry, divorce again, and then go to jail for poisoning your spouse while on vacation, your score would be 370.

Individuals scoring 300 points within a year have an 80 per cent risk of becoming seriously ill, physically or emotionally, in the next year. A score above 150 is followed by a 50 per cent increase, while less than 150 indicates a relatively small amount of life change and, subsequently, low susceptibility to stress-induced illness.

Death of a spouse 100
Divorce 73
Marital separation 65

Death of family member 63
Jail term 63
Personal injury or illness 53
Marriage 50
Fired at work 47
Marital reconciliation 45
Retirement 45
Poor health of family member 44
Pregnancy 40
Sex difficulties 39
Gain a new family member 39
Business readjustment 39
Change in financial situation 38
Death of close friend 37
Change to different line of work 36
Frequent spousal arguments 35
Mortgage over $100,000 31
Foreclosure of loan 30
Change in work responsibilities 29
Son or daughter leaving home 29
Trouble with in-laws 29
Outstanding personal achievement 28
Spouse stops or begins work 26
Change in living conditions 25
Revision of personal habits 24
Trouble with boss 23
Change in work hours/conditions 20
Change in residence 20
Change in schools 20
Change in recreation 19
Change in church activities 19
Change in social activities 18
Mortgage less than $100,000 17
Change in sleeping habits 16

Change in eating habits 15
Vacation 14
Hepburn family vacation 276
Christmas 12
Minor violations of the law 11

Now, by no means is this test all-inclusive, and stress levels may vary depending on circumstance. For example, a $100,000 mortgage may not bother you if, earlier today, you asked your aide to tell your butler to stock your fleet of Leer jets with caviar-producing belugas.

COZYVILLE

Driving into town one day last week, singing lustily as though I'd just been invited to sing baritone with the Mormon Tabernacle Choir, I sped over a rise in the road and was forced to pull over. The viewpoint was one I zoom by every day, but this early December morning a mist rose from the valley and hovered like suspended cotton—partially exposing some buildings and homes, completely erasing others. Rugged snowcapped Olympic mountains loomed in the backdrop, separated from the town by a deep windswept ocean strait. With strains of the Choir's "Shenandoah" waving about my head, I was profoundly awestruck by this Rockwellian moment. The scene was a real-life version of a little porcelain village winter scene that I set up on a coffee table in my home each Christmas. Fluffy, wispy, woolly "snow" wraps securely around miniature houses, shops, a church, and frozen ponds.

This tiny tabletop town awaits Santa or the Savior or grandparents, depending on my mood. But to the chagrin of the inhabitants of what my kids call "Cozyville," it is more often visited by Murphy, my curious, careless hound. Ignoring the detailed precision that has gone into setting up this Christmas village, Murphy rearranges the cotton, leaving wee snowmen, the post office, and a few shocked carolers dangling from his tail.

My reverie was disturbed when I glanced at the car's clock— again I was late for my office. The first patient will be eighty-year-old Irene. Regardless of the reason for her visit, I am certain of one thing she will bring up. Within the first minute or two, she will mention $2,689.47. This number, she has told me each time I've seen her, is the remaining amount that her son owes her from a loan she gave him a few years earlier in order to start a business.

The business struggles, and the debt remains unpaid. But the interest accrues in Irene's craw. She thinks about it day and night. She ruminates and ruminates. Today, once again, she is in my office, wondering why she can't sleep, why she is so easily upset, why she is so anxious and fearful, why she is depressed. She can't begin to appreciate the joy that life offers because she has cluttered her mind with repetitively negative useless worry, as many of us are wont to do.

Are we so preoccupied with minutiae of the past that we spend many of our waking hours, and some sleeping ones, trying to mentally change unchangeable history? The past is over and done with, and all the fretting about it will change nothing. Conversely, we may be so concerned about planning for our future that we are again absorbed, if not consumed, in something other than this very day. Our lives focus so much on how things will get better once we achieve this or obtain that, that we become inattentive to the richness in the present moments and hours of each day.

Are you constantly striving to get somewhere other than where you are? Is fulfillment always just around the corner? Is most of what you do simply a means to an end? And if so, what is that end? The future, when lived at the expense of the present, may lead to worry, anxiety, and unfulfilled stress. Ruminating about the past may lead to regret, sorrow, and depression.

On the way home from work, I gave my vocal cords and the Mormon Tabernacle Choir a break and listened instead to a radio talk show. A birdwatcher was discussing the beauty of ornithology. "How is it," he went on, "that we don't stop to marvel at birds? We ignore the inspiring sight of a soaring hawk, the sweet and happy music of a chirping chickadee, the amazing navigational feats of the Canada goose, the beautiful splashes of color of a mallard or finch, the perfect shape of an egg, the dedication of nesting. Rather, we rush home and turn on our TVs so that we can stare for hours at uninspiring people with uninspiring messages."

To too many of us, life becomes a search for wealth or a search for some form of entertainment or another.

I have started to observe birds. (My hockey team might question my serum "macho" levels at this admission. Fortunately, few of them read.) I do not wish to end up like Irene. So I'm going to wrap this up and go and sit by my little porcelain village and try to place a wee bird on a spire on a church in Cozyville, Murphy permitting.

OPTIMIST CLUB

"A cloudy diagnosis is no match for a sunny disposition."

On the rare occasions I need to make amends on the home front, I find it easiest to buy roses. The florist and I have subsequently become fast friends. "You're late today, doc," she smiles. "Will that be the usual?" Her pleasant face winces as she sweeps the thorns off the stems, pricking her busy fingers yet again. I'm reminded of the adage I heard a thousand times as a child: "Get your fingers out of there!" as well as the other adage, "Instead of complaining that roses have thorns, be grateful that thorns have roses."

TED, FORTY-ONE, had brought his son into the office with an ear infection. But as I glanced at Ted, I noted his eyes were yellowish. I asked how he'd been feeling. "Just fine, doc. The yellow is probably 'cause I've got to find your washroom in a hurry," he joked.

Concerned, I conducted a few tests to discover to my dismay that Ted was breeding pancreatic cancer, a brand of cancer that scares every doctor. When I visited him a few days later in the hospital, he grinned at me and declared he was doing great.

"I have my own TV, the nurses are top notch, and the food is superb."

Either this man was sicker than I thought, or he'd been given an enormous amount of mind-altering drugs. But the nurses were likewise drawn to Ted's upbeat nature, explaining that he never, ever complained. Two months later he was back in hospital, the cancer and the treatment having left him gaunt and wasted.

"Look at this, doc, thinnest I've been in years." As I tried to discuss the gravity of his situation, he interrupted and reminded me, "Everyone has to die sometime, and I've lived a very rich life." A few weeks later he died. Several nurses went to his funeral.

TAKING THE CHART out of the door, I noted my first patient of the day was Ruth. I knew what to expect. Unhappy Ruth would blame someone else for something gone askew, want a CT scan for every sniffle, and complain that she was never well. I didn't recall ever hearing Ruth laugh or even seeing her smile. Constantly beset by a myriad of "problems," she reeked pessimism from every pore. "How are you?" was always met with "Awful."

Did Ted's optimism help him get better? No. Did it affect the way in which he suffered? Without doubt.

Pessimists and those with an attitude of "learned helplessness" not only cope poorly with illness, but they also get more of it. University of Pennsylvania researchers have found that pessimists and their immune systems become more easily depressed. Neurotransmitter action of the pessimist's brain hinders the immune system's NK (natural killer) cells and T cells.

Consequently, the grumps become more ill more often, focus on how much they will suffer, and take longer to heal.

Optimists, in contrast, believe in healthier lifestyles, seek to improve their health, and take bad news as only a temporary setback. Learned helplessness begins in childhood in kids who feel lack of control over their lives. No child should ever hear "Let me do this!" "Hurry up!" "Shut up!" "Useless!" "Stupid!" "That's a poor job!" Such youth acquire learned helplessness and ultimately develop a painful and pessimistic way of seeing the world about them.

IN THE EXTRAORDINARY book *Standing for Something*, the late Gordon B. Hinckley advises that to enhance optimism "... as we go through life, we *accentuate* the positive... look a little deeper for the good... still our voices of insult and sarcasm." He reminds us to "give strength to the voice of hope" and avoid becoming trapped in negative sophistries.

Now, go buy some thorns.

Index